The BUSY MUM'S *gu…* WEIGHT LO…S

on a Budget

BONUS PULL-OUT POSTER FOR YOUR FRIDGE

the healthy Mummy
TEAM
HEALTHY
MUMMY
Rhian27
fridge - Nov2
freezer - Dec1

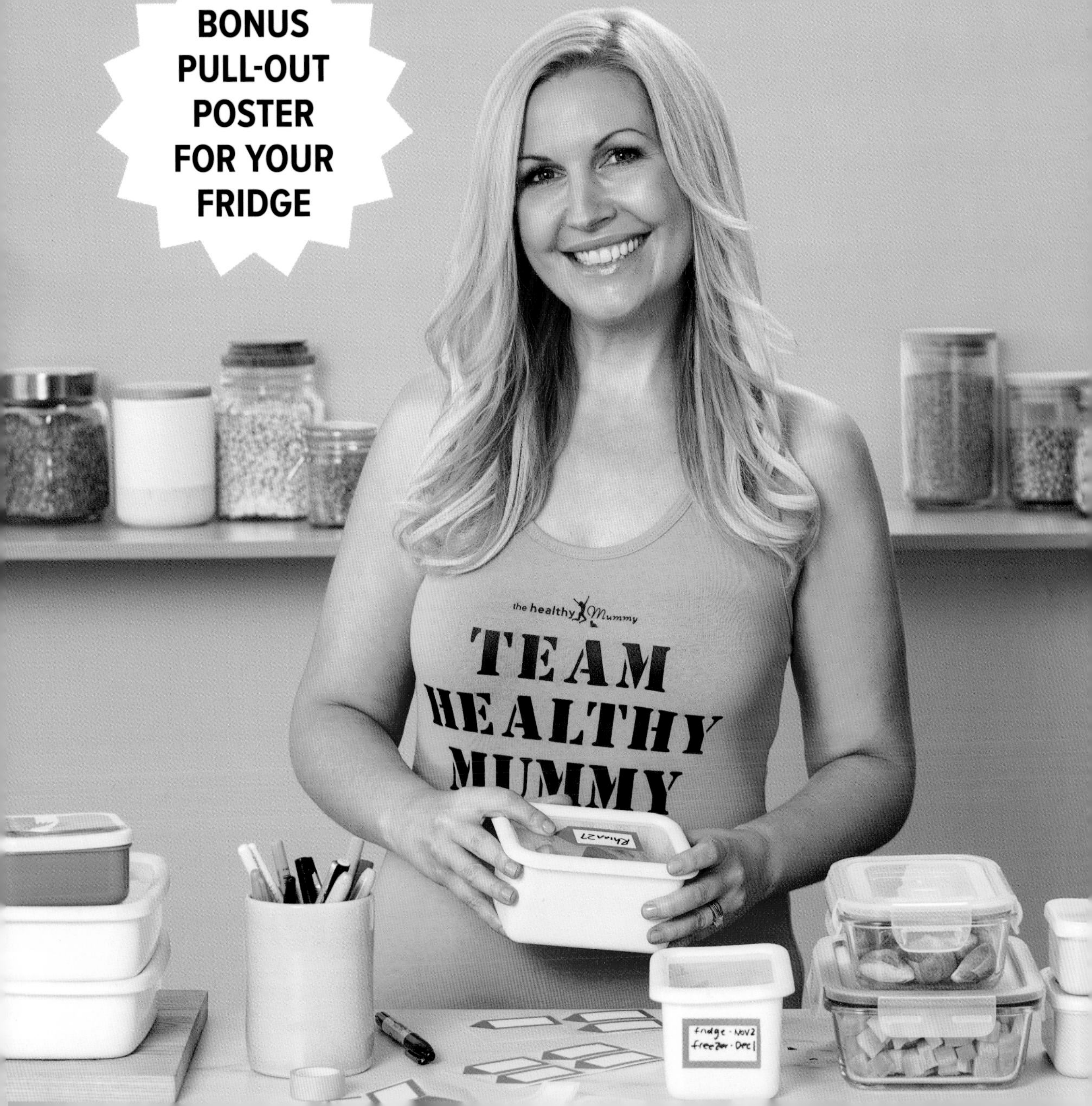

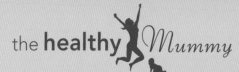
THURSDAY	FRIDAY	SATURDAY	SUNDAY

WEIGHT-LOSS PROGRESS

Keep track of your weight and measurements.

	WAIST (cm)	ARMS (cm)	THIGHS (cm)	HIPS (cm)	WEIGHT (kg)
START					
WEEK 1					
WEEK 2					
WEEK 3					
WEEK 4					
WEEK 5					
WEEK 6					
WEEK 7					
WEEK 8					
WEEK 9					
WEEK 10					
WEEK 11					
WEEK 12					

The Healthy Mummy app can help you keep track of your progress. Go to healthymummy.com to access.

MY GOALS FOR THE MONTH

MY REWARDS

FREEZING FOOD

INGREDIENT/DISH	RECOMMENDED STORAGE TIME (MAX)	NOTES
Chopped veggies (both raw and cooked)	1 month	This timeline is driven by food quality rather than food safety. Only freeze vegetables that you are going to cook or reheat when thawed, not eat raw.
Cooked muffins/cakes	2–6 months	This timeline is driven by food quality rather than food safety.
Cooked pasta	1–2 months	This timeline is driven by food quality rather than food safety.
Cooked rice	1–2 months	You can store cooked rice for longer than 1–2 months but the freezing process will affect the quality. After thawing, always reheat to steaming before eating.
Meat	3–6 months	You can store meat for longer than 3–6 months but the freezing process will affect the quality. Freeze meat before the use-by date and after thawing use within 24 hours. Thaw in the fridge or microwave; don't leave out on the bench.
Poultry	6–12 months	You can store poultry for longer than 6–12 months but the freezing process will affect the quality. Freeze poultry before the use-by date and after thawing use within 24 hours. Thaw in the fridge or microwave; don't leave out on the bench.

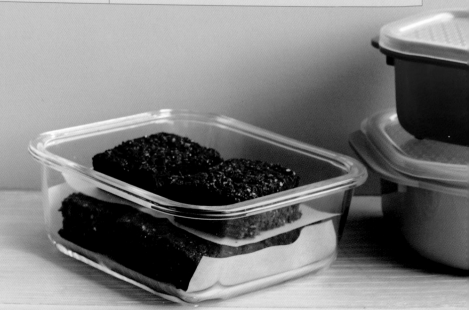

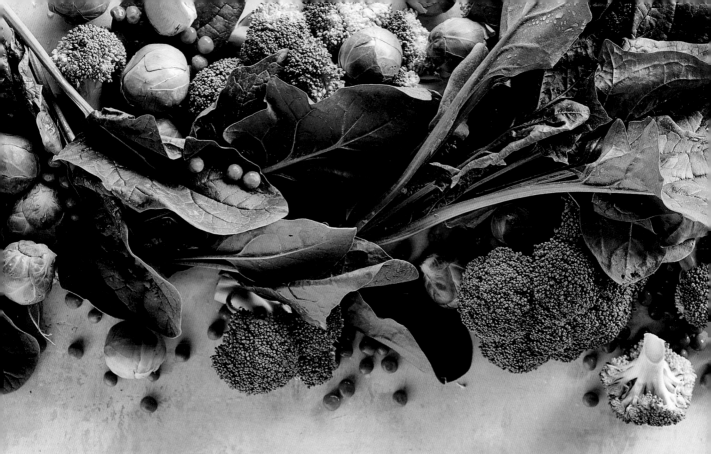

The BUSY MUM'S guide to WEIGHT LOSS
on a Budget

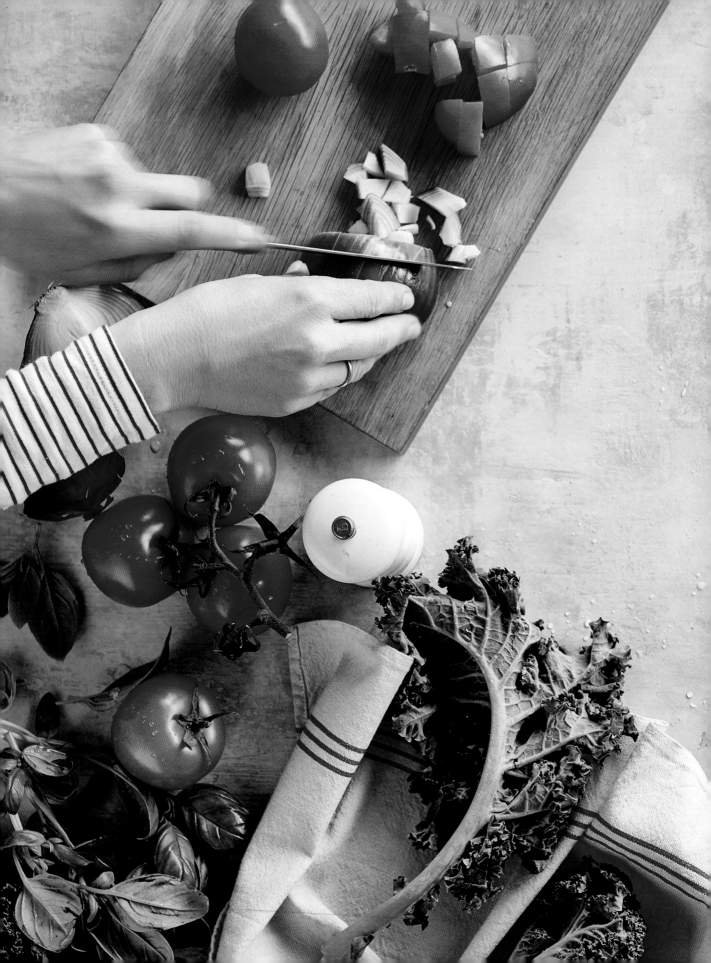

Still want more?

Access bonus book content, including exercises, meal plans and extra recipes, at **healthymummy.com/busy-mums-budget-guide**

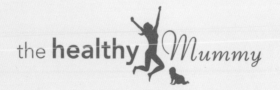

WEEKLY MEAL PLANNER

	MONDAY	TUESDAY	WEDNESDAY
BREAKFAST			
CALORIES			
MORNING SNACK			
CALORIES			
LUNCH			
CALORIES			
AFTERNOON SNACK			
CALORIES			
DINNER			
CALORIES			
EVENING SNACK			
CALORIES			
TOTAL DAILY CALORIES			

WEEKLY SHOPPING LIST

VEGETABLES

DAIRY

FRUIT

MEAT, POULTRY AND FISH

FRESH HERBS

DRY GOODS

FOOD STORAGE GUIDE

Make bulk cooking and meal planning easy with our recommended food-storage times for the fridge and freezer.

REFRIGERATING FOOD

INGREDIENT/DISH	RECOMMENDED STORAGE TIME (MAX)	NOTES
Chopped raw veggies	2 days	Pre-chopped veggies that are going to be eaten raw should be eaten within 2 days to prevent dehydration and bacteria. If you are going to cook the veggies, they can be refrigerated for an extra day or two.
Cooked meats	2–4 days	Store in an airtight container to eat cold or reheat to steaming.
Cooked muffins/cakes	3–4 days	Muffins and cakes are best stored in the freezer to prevent dehydration.
Cooked pasta	3 days	Store in an airtight container to eat cold or reheat to steaming. Don't store any secondary leftovers.
Cooked poultry	3 days	Store in an airtight container to eat cold or reheat to steaming.
Cooked rice	2–3 days	Lay flat in a container to cool quickly as rice is susceptible to bacteria build up. Reheat to steaming and don't store any secondary leftovers.
Cooked seafood	2 days	Store in an airtight container to eat cold or reheat to steaming.

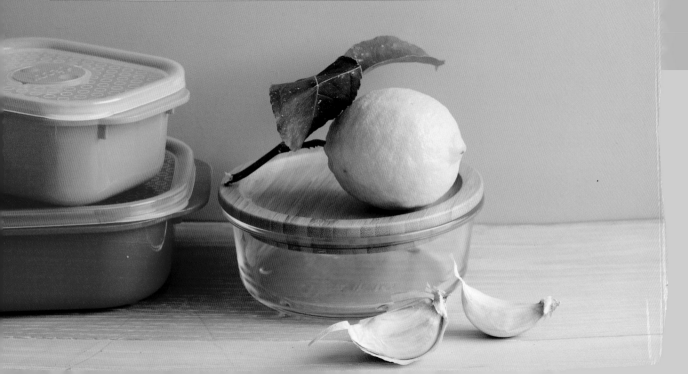

The BUSY MUM'S guide to WEIGHT LOSS

on a Budget

Rhian Allen

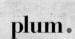 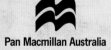

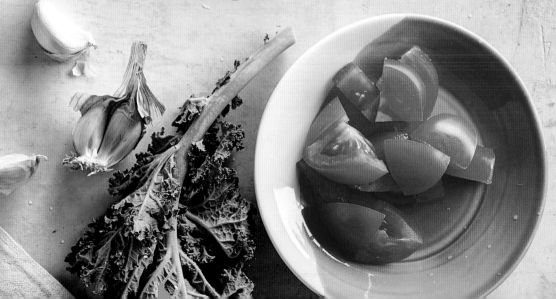

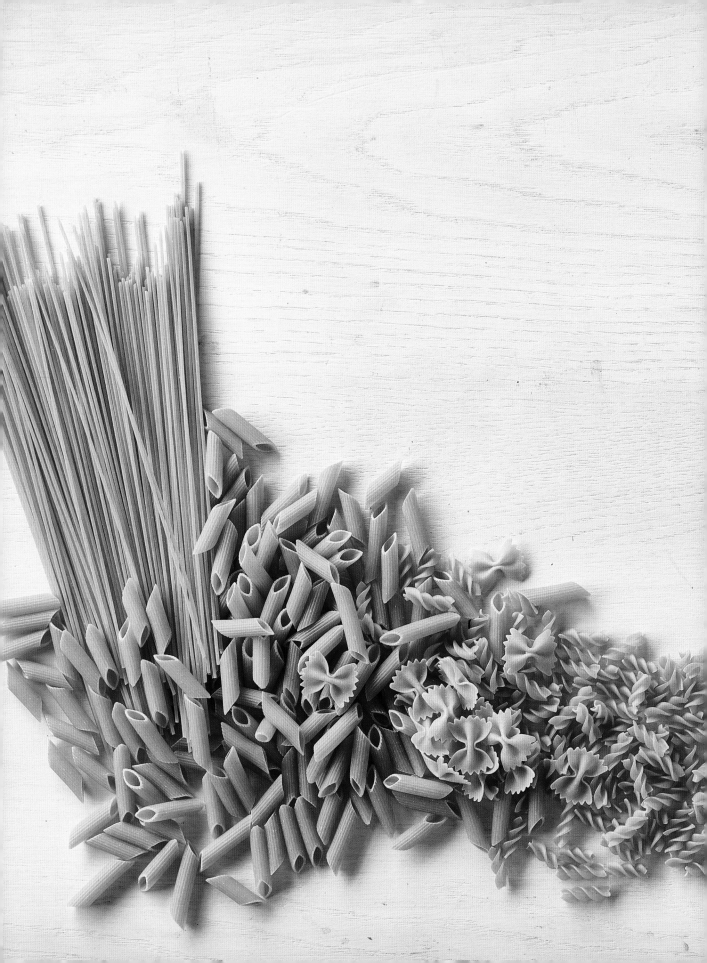

Contents

Introduction 7

Bulk Cooking 36

BREAKFAST 43

SMOOTHIES 83

SALADS & LIGHT MEALS 99

SOUPS 125

PASTA, NOODLES & RICE 133

STOVETOP 149

BAKES 173

SNACKS 203

SWEETS & DESSERTS 219

Thanks 249

Index 251

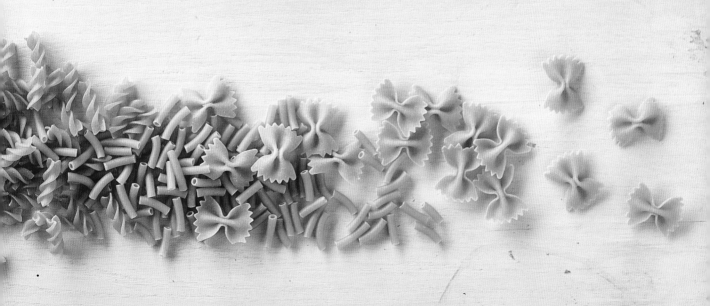

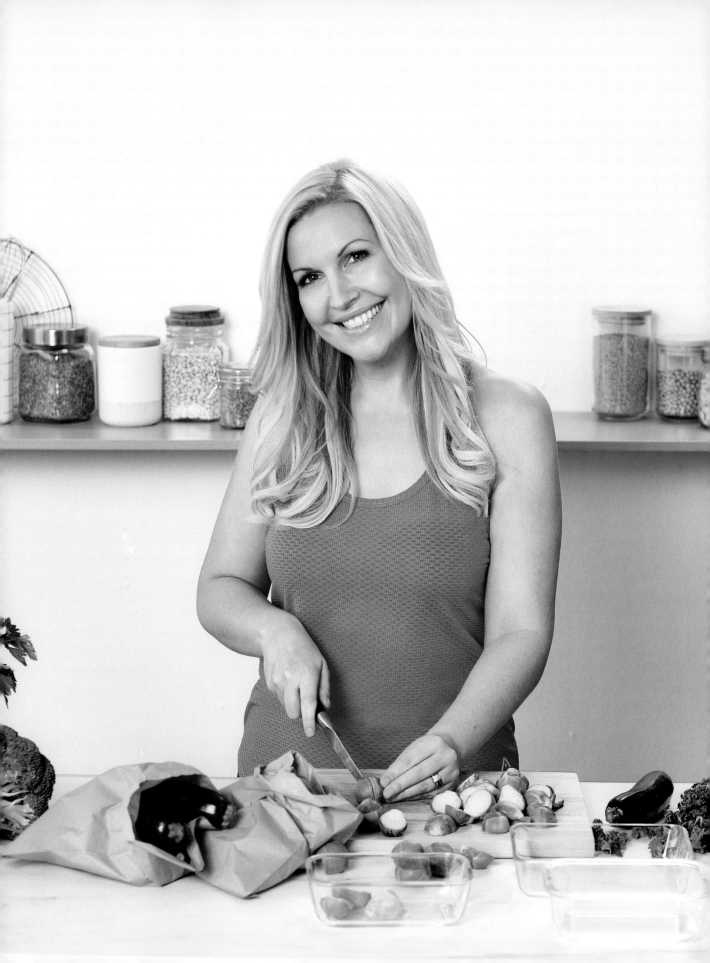

INTRODUCTION

As a mum of two, I understand that motherhood is demanding, and that trying to find time for yourself can be difficult. So, in 2010, I started healthymummy.com as a holistic and national support system to help mums to shape up and get healthy after having a baby.

At The Healthy Mummy, we create healthy eating plans and products to empower mums to live a healthier life. Our practical advice, healthy recipes and customised meal and exercise plans are all family *and* budget friendly. We are growing every day, and I'm proud to say we're currently the biggest mums-only healthy-eating and lifestyle program and support network globally.

Putting ourselves first is the key to a physically and mentally healthy lifestyle for us mums, and our families – and I'm here to prove to you that setting and reaching goals to put you and your health top of mind doesn't need to be difficult or expensive.

The Busy Mum's Guide to Weight Loss on a Budget is loaded with tips and tricks on how to reach your healthy lifestyle goals without spending a fortune. You won't find suggestions for expensive gym memberships, personal trainers or costly pre-prepared meal services in here. What you *will* find are my favourite budget- and family-friendly recipes, plus advice on how you can become the best version of yourself – all without breaking the bank.

Look out for Team Tips throughout the book! They're real feedback from women who are part of The Healthy Mummy community. They include tips from both working and stay-at-home mums, and will help you start and stick to your new lifestyle.

Let's get healthy!

Rhian

Founder, The Healthy Mummy
healthymummy.com

LOSE WEIGHT ON A BUDGET

Eating healthy food can be expensive: buying takeaway, ready-made or processed healthy-eating options costs a lot more than making healthy food yourself – and they don't always fill you up for very long, or provide you with the nutrients you need for a healthy lifestyle.

Losing weight can be simple, if you eat a balanced diet, watch portion sizes, stay hydrated and get active more regularly. Exercise is a fundamental part of your weight-loss journey and The Healthy Mummy has many budget-friendly exercises you can do from the comfort of your own home. Go to healthymummy.com/busy-mums-budget-guide for some quick workouts to get you started.

Budget healthy eating is the key! It's a no-nonsense skill set that involves:

- choosing fresh, seasonal ingredients
- shopping and cooking in bulk
- meal planning
- reducing food waste.

We're here to help you learn these skills and reach your weight-loss goals, while sticking to your budget.

Team Tip

'Make double, triple or quadruple amounts of your dinner recipe each night and freeze it. That's how I started. Always having a freezer full of meals and snacks absolutely keeps me on track!'

– KAITIE, LOST 21 KG

START WITH A QUICK CALCULATION

On a journey to weight loss, it's important to know where you're starting from and where you want to go. Working out your BMR (Basal Metabolic Rate) will tell you how many calories your body needs to function, depending on your personal information such as age, height and weight. Once you know your BMR, you can work out how many calories you should consume each day to reach your weight-loss goals.

Keep these points in mind:

- Always stick to a sensible daily calorie level, because eating below your BMR can prevent you from losing weight, as your body goes into starvation mode and stores energy to keep you functioning.
- Choose nutrient-dense foods to ensure you are providing your body with essential vitamins and minerals for healthy living.
- Never drop your daily calorie intake below 1200 for women and 1800 for men.

FIND YOUR CALORIE NUMBER

Use the formula below to work out your BMR calorie requirements:

Women
BMR = 655 + (9.6 × your weight in kg) + (1.9 × your height in cm) – (4.7 × your age in years)

Men
BMR = 67 + (13.75 × your weight in kg) + (5 × your height in cm) – (6.8 × your age in years)

Once you have your BMR figure, you can work out how many calories you need to consume each day to *maintain your current weight*, depending on how active you are.

Multiply your BMR by the activity level below that most suits your current lifestyle:

- If you do little or no exercise, multiply your BMR by 1.1.
- If you do light exercise or sports 1–3 days per week, multiply your BMR by 1.275.
- If you do moderate exercise or sports 3–5 days per week, multiply your BMR by 1.35.
- If you do hard exercise or sports 6–7 days per week, multiply your BMR by 1.525.

DROP THE EXCESS

Take the BMR figure you now have and reduce it by 10–15 per cent.

This will give you the average number of calories you should consume each day to reach your weight-loss goals. Remember, this figure is just a guide and shouldn't rule your life. If you feel hungry, eat more – choosing healthy options, of course! If you feel too full trying to reach your daily calorie figure, reduce your portion sizes or miss a snack between main meals.

If you're breastfeeding, allow an extra 500 calories per day on top of your target calorie needs for weight loss, as you're using more energy for milk production.

SET GOALS AND REWARDS

Now you've done the maths, set two or three specific goals and rewards to help you reach your weight-loss target and give them a realistic timeframe.

Goals should be SMART: Specific, Measurable, Attainable, Relevant and Time-bound; for example, 'I am going to lose 5 kg in 8 weeks' rather than 'I want to be slimmer'.

Rewards should be simple and not food based, such as a copy of your favourite magazine or a new nail polish for achieving small goals, such as exercising every day for a week.

Plan larger rewards (such as a trip to a day spa, a new outfit or a night out with your partner) for reaching the bigger goals, such as hitting a goal weight.

Regularly check in with your goal achievements, adjusting them to suit changes you've made and reward yourself, even for the little successes. The weekly meal planner poster at the front of this book has a section to record your goals and rewards.

Top tip for goal achievement

An inspiration board can be a really powerful visual tool to help you reach your goals. Fill it with images and words that say and show what you're trying to achieve, and put it up somewhere you'll see it every day.

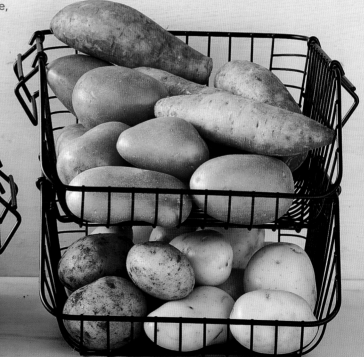

MEAL PLANNING

Meal planning is probably *the* most important thing you can do
to reach your weight-loss goals and stay within your budget.

BECOME A PLANNING PRO!

You'll soon grow to love meal planning. Why?
Meal planning:

- gets you ready for the weeks and even months ahead
- stocks up your freezer
- saves time in the kitchen
- means you can buy and cook in bulk and take advantage of specials to save money.

Following a meal plan is the key to weight-loss success, as you're much less likely to fill up on unhealthy snacks, order takeaway or make the wrong food choices.

MAKE MEAL PLANNING SIMPLE

Plan

Allow time in your day to meal plan every week/fortnight/month.

Check

What leftovers/frozen meals do you already have? Incorporate these into your plan to use them up. Check your pantry and plan meals around food that you already have available.

Repeat

Make meals in bulk and assign them to a couple of nights a week, or freeze and repeat your meal plan every fortnight.

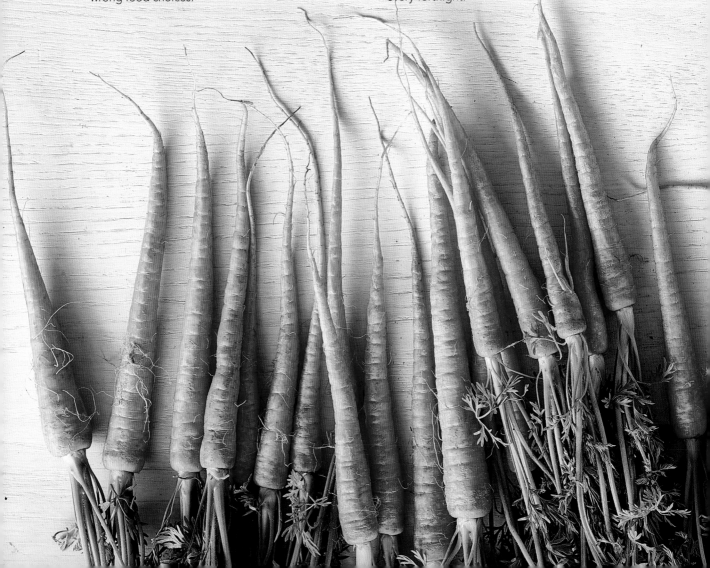

Keep it simple

Choose one or two easy-to-prepare, healthy breakfast recipes for each week and then make extra portions of your dinners to reheat for lunch the next day.

Snack smart

Assign a few healthy snacks to make in bulk each time and have plenty of inexpensive, healthy options on hand as well, such as fresh fruit and veggies, wholegrain crackers, nuts, natural yoghurt etc.

Stick to it!

This is the most important bit. There's no point in writing a meal plan and shopping for the recipes and then not following it. Choosing healthy recipes you know you and your family will enjoy will make it easier to stick to.

We've created a sample weekly meal plan on pp. 14–15 using recipes from this book to help you get started. Or you can make your own using the weekly meal planner poster.

Handy hints

- Feel free to swap recipes in or out of our sample meal plan to suit your family's tastes.

- Try to repurpose leftovers into new meals.

- Include meals that are made with ingredients you already have.

Team Tip

'I don't have time to make a different lunch every day before I rush out the door to work. So, instead, I make up the same lunch for the whole week and have a few different snack options to mix things up.'

– ANGELA

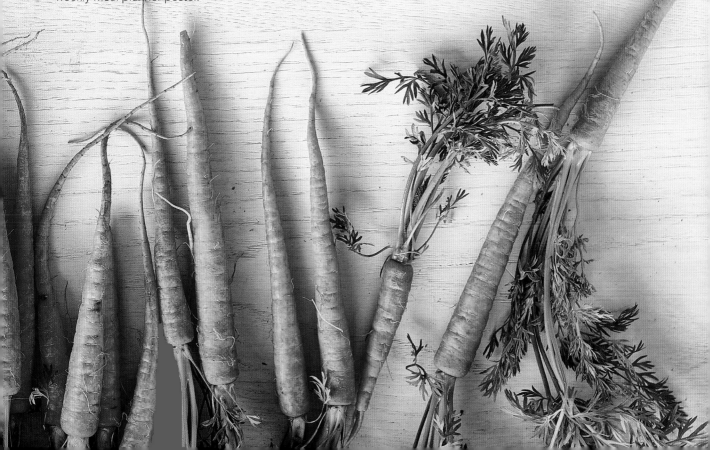

PLAN MEALS ON A BUDGET

Choose cuts and carbs

Choose healthy, family-friendly recipes for your meal plans that use cheaper cuts of meat (think slow-cooked curries, stews, pasta sauces etc.), plus plenty of complex carbohydrates and vegetables to bulk them out.

Bulk up your meals

Choose meals that use budget-friendly basics, such as wholegrain pasta, brown rice and legumes. For example, add some canned lentils to your bolognese sauce to increase the fibre content, make the meal go further and, in turn, save money.

Go vegetarian

Meat is usually the most expensive part of a meal, so include more vegetable-based dishes to help you to stick to your budget and increase your intake of healthy nutrients. Lots of nutrient-dense vegetables (such as sweet potato, beetroot and leafy greens) make great additions to meals and they will also keep you feeling fuller for longer, meaning you're less likely to overeat.

Boost the base

Bulk-cook time-saving base recipes that can be turned into different options for your meal plan; for example, a bolognese sauce could become the base for a meat pie, chilli con carne or a filling for baked potatoes. Having a few of these in your repertoire makes it easier to cook in bulk, saving time and money (see Bulk Cooking, p. 36).

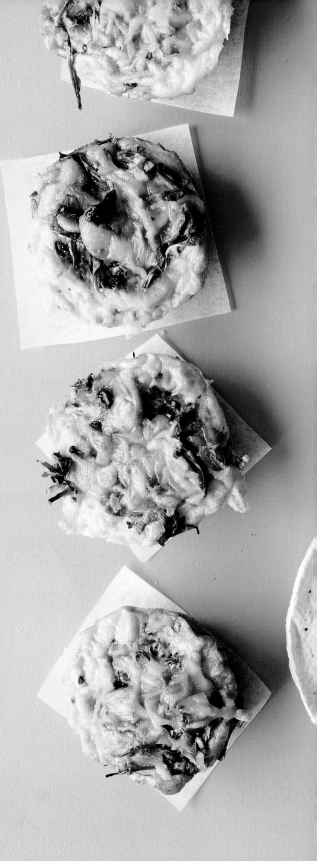

> *Team Tip*
>
> *'I'm out of the house all week, so I'm all about not doing something for a single purpose! I make the main component for most meals and then repurpose it for something else. So spag bol turns into a chilli or lasagne. If I'm making hard-boiled eggs, I do egg sandwiches, and so on. It saves so much time!'*
>
> **– DEB**

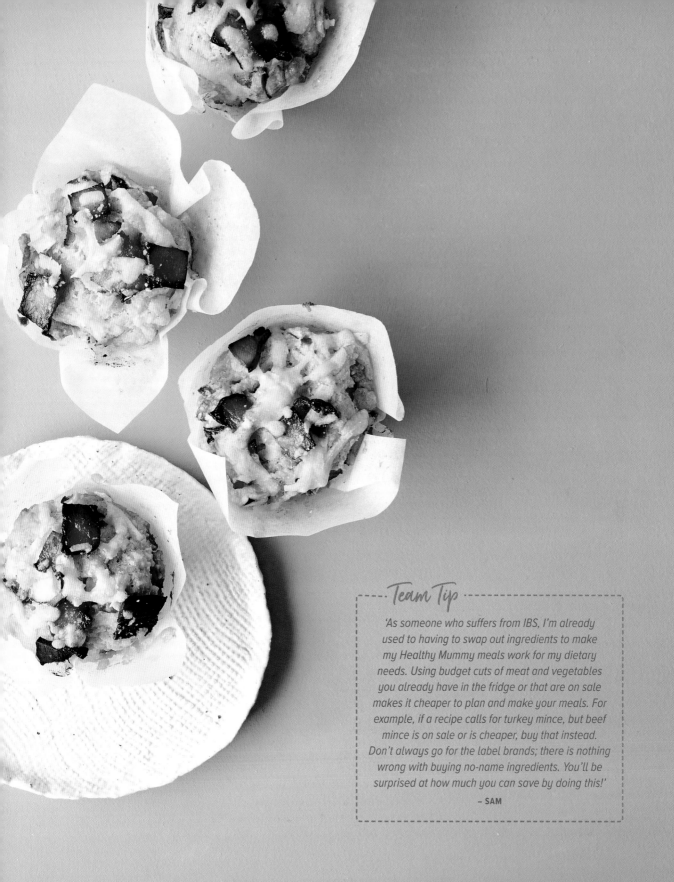

---···· *Team Tip* ·····---

*'As someone who suffers from IBS, I'm already
used to having to swap out ingredients to make
my Healthy Mummy meals work for my dietary
needs. Using budget cuts of meat and vegetables
you already have in the fridge or that are on sale
makes it cheaper to plan and make your meals. For
example, if a recipe calls for turkey mince, but beef
mince is on sale or is cheaper, buy that instead.
Don't always go for the label brands; there is nothing
wrong with buying no-name ingredients. You'll be
surprised at how much you can save by doing this!'*

– SAM

SAMPLE 7-DAY MEAL PLAN

Use any of the recipes in this book to create your own meal plan (using the pull-out weekly meal planner provided!), but here is a sample plan to get you started. Please see overleaf for a shopping list.

	DAY 1	DAY 2	DAY 3
BREAKFAST	PEANUT BUTTER GRANOLA P. 52	APPLE AND BLUEBERRY CORNBREAD P. 46	CORN AND HAM BREAKFAST SLICE P. 77
Calories	304	334	325
Cost per serve	$0.68	$1.33	$1.47
MORNING SNACK	BEETROOT, MINT AND CASHEW DIP P. 207	CUP OF HERBAL TEA AND ¼ CUP ALMONDS	BEETROOT, MINT AND CASHEW DIP P. 207
Calories	149	187	149
Cost per serve	$1.03	$0.49	$1.03
LUNCH	CHICKEN CAESAR WRAP P. 119	SLOW-COOKED TORTELLINI AND VEGETABLE SOUP P. 126	HIDDEN VEG BOLOGNESE POTATO P. 197
Calories	307	326	383
Cost per serve	$2.00	$1.74	$1.80
AFTERNOON SNACK	CUP OF HERBAL TEA AND 1 LARGE APPLE (200 G)	CAJUN CHICKEN MEATBALLS P. 215	CUP OF HERBAL TEA AND 1 LARGE APPLE (200 G)
Calories	117	167	117
Cost per serve	$0.69	$1.20	$0.69
DINNER	SAUSAGE AND VEGETABLE PASTA BAKE P. 136	ZOODLES WITH HIDDEN VEG BOLOGNESE P. 144	CAJUN CHICKEN PIZZA P. 189
Calories	455	241	380
Cost per serve	$1.55	$1.92	$2.22
EVENING SNACK	PEANUT BUTTER AND CHOCOLATE BROWNIE BITE P. 226	½ CUP REDUCED-FAT GREEK YOGHURT, WITH 1 TABLESPOON SHREDDED COCONUT AND 1 TEASPOON HONEY	PEANUT BUTTER AND CHOCOLATE BROWNIE BITE P. 226
Calories	145	191	145
Cost per serve	$0.35	$0.61	$0.35
TOTAL DAILY CALORIES	1477	1446	1499
DAILY COST PER PERSON	$6.30	$7.29	$7.56

DAY 4	DAY 5	DAY 6	DAY 7
APPLE AND BLUEBERRY CORNBREAD P. 46	**PEANUT BUTTER GRANOLA P. 52**	**CORN AND HAM BREAKFAST SLICE P. 77**	**APPLE AND BLUEBERRY CORNBREAD P. 46**
334	304	325	334
$1.33	$0.68	$1.47	$1.33
BEETROOT, MINT AND CASHEW DIP P. 207	**CAJUN CHICKEN MEATBALLS P. 215**	**CUP OF HERBAL TEA AND ¼ CUP ALMONDS**	**BEETROOT, MINT AND CASHEW DIP P. 207**
149	167	187	149
$1.03	$1.20	$0.49	$1.03
GREEK TUNA SALAD P. 116	**HAM, SPINACH AND FETA PIZZA P. 189**	**SLOW-COOKED TORTELLINI AND VEGETABLE SOUP P. 126**	**CHICKEN AND JALAPENO POPPERS WITH GUACAMOLE P. 182**
199	303	326	331
$1.50	$2.50	$1.74	$2.03
CAJUN CHICKEN MEATBALLS P. 215	**CUP OF HERBAL TEA AND ¼ CUP ALMONDS**	**CAJUN CHICKEN MEATBALLS P. 215**	**CUP OF HERBAL TEA AND 1 LARGE APPLE (200 G)**
167	187	167	117
$1.20	$0.49	$1.20	$0.69
SAUSAGE AND VEGETABLE PASTA BAKE P. 136	**HIDDEN VEG BOLOGNESE PIE P. 196**	**PUMPKIN AND FETA TART P. 188**	**SPICED CHICKPEA BOWL P. 108**
455	347	310	410
$1.55	$1.22	$1.15	$1.95
PEANUT BUTTER AND CHOCOLATE BROWNIE BITE P. 226	**½ CUP REDUCED-FAT GREEK YOGHURT, WITH 1 TABLESPOON SHREDDED COCONUT AND 1 TEASPOON HONEY**	**PEANUT BUTTER AND CHOCOLATE BROWNIE BITE P. 226**	**PEANUT BUTTER AND CHOCOLATE BROWNIE BITE P. 226**
145	191	145	145
$0.35	$0.61	$0.35	$0.35
1449	1499	1460	1486
$6.96	$6.70	$6.40	$7.38

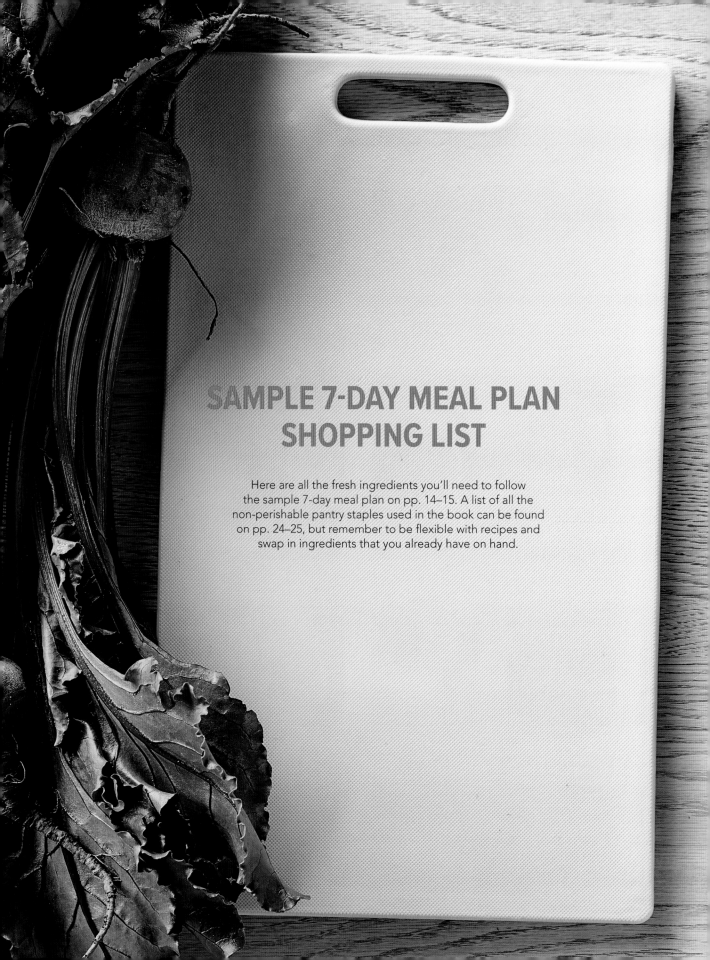

SAMPLE 7-DAY MEAL PLAN SHOPPING LIST

Here are all the fresh ingredients you'll need to follow
the sample 7-day meal plan on pp. 14–15. A list of all the
non-perishable pantry staples used in the book can be found
on pp. 24–25, but remember to be flexible with recipes and
swap in ingredients that you already have on hand.

Vegetables

Baby beetroot 4
Baby spinach leaves 300 g
Beans, green 120 g
Broccoli 100 g
Cabbage, red 100 g
Capsicums, red 2
Carrots 15
Celery stalks 5
Cos lettuce 15 g
Cucumber, Lebanese 1
Garlic cloves 13
Kale leaves 30 g
Mixed lettuce leaves 120 g
Onion, red 1
Onions, brown 3
Potatoes 4
Pumpkin 960 g
Rocket leaves 90 g
Spring onion 1
Sweet potato 1
Tomatoes 3
Zucchini 8

Fruit

Apples 4
Avocado 1
Blueberries 260 g (or use frozen)
Lemon 1
Lime 1
Medjool dates 180 g

Fresh herbs

Basil 1 bunch
Coriander 1 bunch
Flat-leaf parsley 1 bunch
Mint 1 bunch

Meat, poultry and eggs

Beef mince, lean 480 g
Chicken breast fillets 1.4 kg
Free-range eggs 17
Ham, lean, smoked 260 g (13 slices)
Pork mince, lean 480 g
Sausages of choice, lean 560 g

Dairy

Cheddar, reduced-fat 600 g
Cream cheese, light 130 g
Feta, reduced-fat 160 g
Milk of choice, reduced-fat 625 ml
Parmesan, grated 85 g
Sour cream, light 65 g
Yoghurt, reduced-fat plain Greek 855 g

Breads, grains, cereals and nuts

Mountain bread wrap, wholemeal 1
Pita bread, wholemeal, medium 10
Tortillas, mini 8

Other

Fresh spinach and ricotta tortellini 400 g

Team Tip

'I love roasting a whole tray of veggies on a Sunday and turning them into multiple dishes throughout the week: frittata, salad, pasta or as a side with meat or fish.' – RACHAEL

BULK SHOPPING

Once you have your meal plan prepared, organise your shopping to ensure it's as budget friendly as possible.

The two key things for budget-friendly shopping are to assess what items you already have and to write a shopping list that you will stick to.

Start by preparing a shopping list to match the recipes in your meal plan. Then do a pantry, fridge and freezer inventory to see what ingredients you already have. Many people are surprised at how many cans of tomatoes, bags of rice or jars of dried herbs they have hiding in their cupboards!

When assessing the ingredients you already have, see if you can make any swaps in the recipes you're planning to prepare. It's easy to swap fruit, veggies, grains, legumes, cheese and even protein in many recipes. Just because a stir-fry recipe calls for broccoli, carrot and capsicum doesn't mean you can't make it with zucchini, corn and beans. Using up what you already have available will save you lots at the checkout.

Every week, schedule in time for meal planning, preparing your shopping list, and doing the shopping. Having a set day to do these tasks will help to make them part of your routine, avoiding the need for sporadic visits to the supermarket that could blow your budget.

All of the recipes in this book feature a 'cost per serve' figure, which all come in at under $2.50 per serve. These costs per serve figures are calculated based on the cost of mid-range products found in all major supermarkets. Buying in bulk and/or home-brand products may further reduce the cost per serve.

TOP TIPS FOR BUDGET SHOPPING

Stay seasonal and local

You'll pay a premium to buy ingredients out of season or shipped from a distance. When planning your weekly menu, swap fresh fruit and vegetables that aren't in season for ones that are, or buy them frozen. When an in-season ingredient is on special (for example, tomatoes or stone fruits in summer), buy them in bulk and turn them into a homemade tomato sauce or stewed fruit, to freeze and use throughout the year.

Shop online

This will save you time and can make it easier to stick to your budget, as you generally only buy what's on your list and are less likely to be tempted by impulse purchases. Most major supermarkets offer free click and collect services, so you don't have to pay delivery fees.

Don't shop hungry

You may be tempted to add extra items to your trolley that your tummy is saying you want!

Buy in bulk

If you have the space in your freezer, buy bulk meats and frozen foods when they're on special, to freeze in smaller portions. There are lots of non-perishable pantry staples, such as flours, grains, rice and canned goods, that are also great to buy in bulk when on special.

Shop around

Prices vary hugely across different supermarkets. If you have access to a wholesale supermarket you could shop with a friend and share the cost of buying non-perishable items in bulk. Visiting your local farmers' market or greengrocer can also ensure you get fresh, local produce.

Speak up

Don't be afraid to ask for a discount if buying in bulk – lots of butchers and fishmongers will offer a bulk-buy price. Store in your freezer or share a bulk pack with a friend or relative.

Use price per unit

Manufacturers pay a premium to have their products displayed in a certain area of the supermarket, so just because something is on special doesn't mean it's the cheapest item of its kind. All price tags in a supermarket should include a 'price per unit' or 'price per 100 g'. Compare these to find the most budget-friendly item.

Team Tip

'I shop two or three times a week so all my fruit and veg are fresh, which means I'm more likely to stay the course. I also pack almonds and an apple in sandwich bags and pop them in the fridge for an easy grab and make up little trail mixes, so I always have something healthy to eat on the run.'

— KRYSTAL

Check the chiller

Some frozen fruit and vegetables actually contain more nutrients than fresh because they're packed as soon as they're picked. If frozen items are cheaper, use these instead of fresh.

Avoid processed foods

These items contain more additives, salt, sugar and preservatives than fresh foods, and they cost more. Where possible, make homemade versions to save money and improve your nutritional intake.

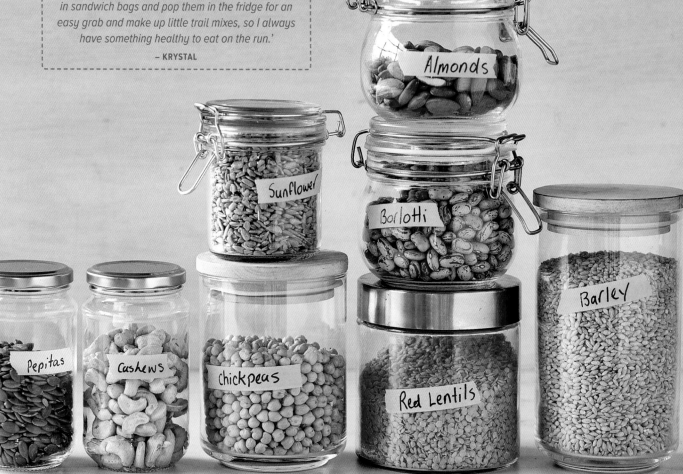

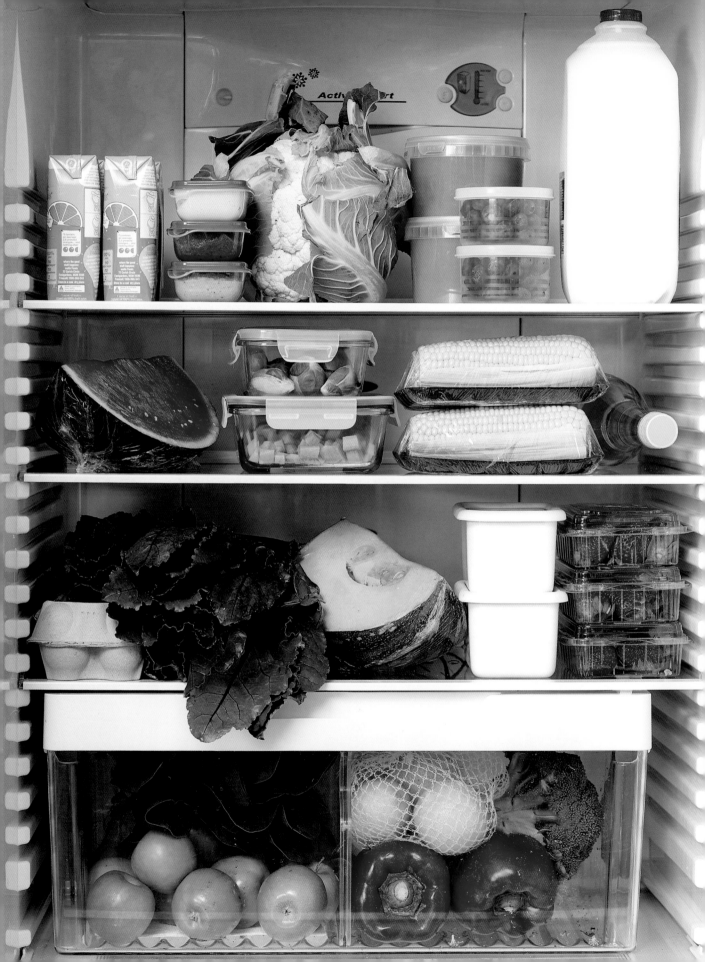

STOCK UP ON STAPLE INGREDIENTS

When you see the following ingredients on sale, buy them in bulk if you have the space to store them. These budget-friendly ingredients are great to have on hand if you're trying to lose weight and maintain a healthy lifestyle.

- **Canned or frozen fruits and vegetables:** with no added salt and canned fruit in juice, not syrup.

- **Rolled oats:** home-brand options are often the same as the premium versions but less than half the price.

- **Canned fish, such as tuna and salmon:** great to add to a pasta sauce, mix with steamed veggies, or add to a sandwich or salad.

- **Canned legumes:** a much cheaper source of protein than meat, add these to pasta sauces, curries or stews to bulk them up.

- **Brown rice and wholegrain pasta:** loaded with fibre, they'll keep you feeling fuller for longer and are a great way to bulk up meals. Buy rice in bulk, not in microwaveable packs, to save money. To make life easier during the busy working week, you can pre-cook brown rice and store it in the fridge for 2–3 days or freeze for up to 2 months, to use later in meals. Just be sure to reheat it to steaming before use.

- **Dried herbs and spices:** cheaper than fresh and will last a lot longer. Buy them on special to gradually build up a good range of options to give your meals flavour.

- **UHT milk:** very handy to use in baking or cooking. Having a few cartons in the pantry will take care of any last-minute needs.

- **Eggs:** a great source of protein, containing healthy fats and essential amino acids. Scramble them for breakfast, hard-boil them for a healthy snack, add them to sandwiches, or use them to make a cost-effective omelette for dinner.

- **Cheaper cuts of meat:** flank, chuck or blade instead of rump or rib-eye steak; or chicken thigh instead of breast. These are ideal to make bulk recipes, such as stews, curries and slow-cooked meals. Trim off any excess fat before cooking.

- **Bananas:** the ultimate 'packaged' food. Add them to smoothies, lunchboxes and your favourite baking recipes. Peeling and freezing overripe bananas and then blitzing them in a food processor makes the best healthy 'ice cream'. Bananas are loaded with potassium, as well as other minerals and vitamins to keep you healthy and fill you up at a low price.

- **Sweet potatoes:** a low-cost veggie that's really nutrient dense. Add to stews and curries to bulk them up, or roast them first and add to salads and pizzas for a cheap nutrition hit.

Team Tip

'Picking meals that use a cheaper cut of meat helps a lot with my budget. Bulk minced meat, sausages or chicken thighs are easy to cook with and really help keep the cost down.' – **SARAH**

Team Tip

'I use the same ingredients for the week, so if we're having something in one meal we will have it in two or three meals. This way I can buy in bulk and save on money and time.' – **RAE**

Swap and Save

Save money by making these simple ingredient swaps:

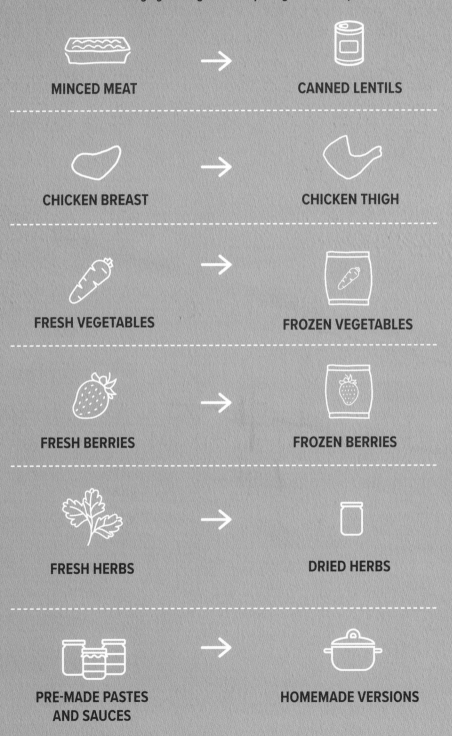

MINCED MEAT → CANNED LENTILS

CHICKEN BREAST → CHICKEN THIGH

FRESH VEGETABLES → FROZEN VEGETABLES

FRESH BERRIES → FROZEN BERRIES

FRESH HERBS → DRIED HERBS

PRE-MADE PASTES AND SAUCES → HOMEMADE VERSIONS

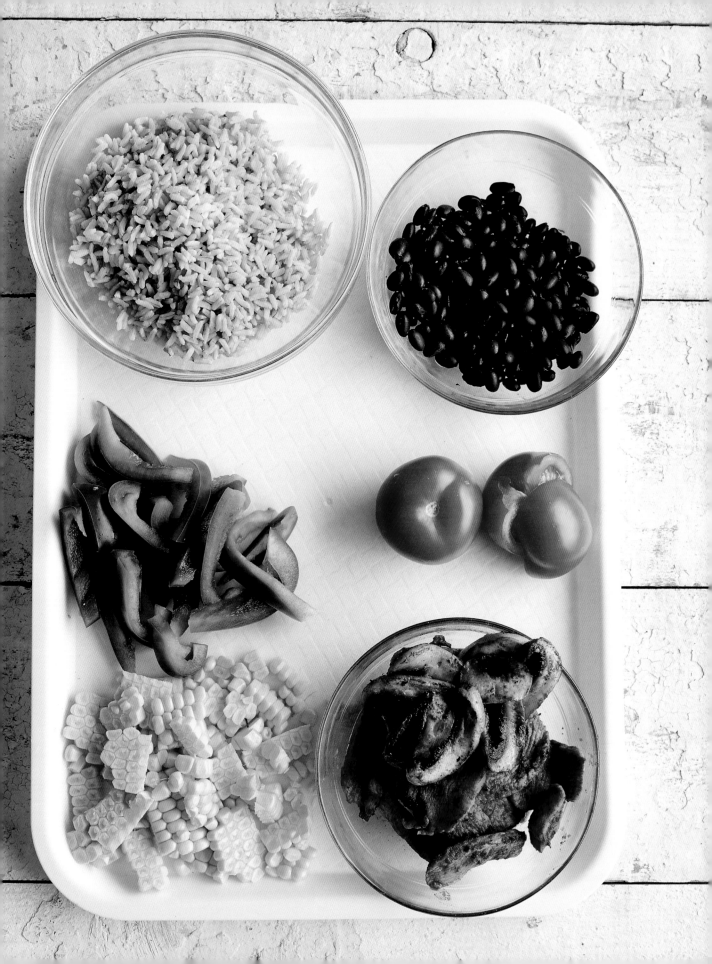

PANTRY STAPLES

The following list includes all the non-perishable items used in the recipes in this book. Of course, you don't need to have all of these items on hand – think of it as a guide – but having a well-stocked pantry makes eating healthily on a budget so much easier.

Cans and packaged food

Apricots, dried
Baking powder
Beetroot slices, canned
Bicarbonate of soda
Black beans, canned
Cacao nibs
Cacao powder
Cannellini beans, canned
Chickpeas, canned
Chocolate, dark (70% cocoa solids)
Coconut cream
Coconut sugar
Coconut water
Coffee, instant
Corn chips, plain
Corn kernels, canned
Cranberries, dried
Dates
Gelatine, powdered
Jalapeno chillies, pickled
Kidney beans, canned
Lentils, brown, canned
Lentils, brown, dried
Pappadums, mini
Peas, frozen
Peppermint extract
Pineapple, canned
Puff pastry, reduced-fat, frozen
Rice paper sheets
Smoothie powders (chocolate, strawberry and vanilla)
Stevia, liquid
Stevia, powder
Stock, salt-reduced, beef
Stock, salt-reduced, chicken
Stock, salt-reduced, vegetable
Taco shells
Teabags, herbal
Tomatoes, whole peeled and diced, canned
Tuna in spring water, canned
Vanilla extract

Grains, cereals, nuts and seeds

Almond meal
Almonds, flaked
Almonds, whole
Breadcrumbs, dried, wholemeal
Cashews, unsalted
Chia seeds
Coconut flour
Coconut, desiccated
Coconut, shredded
Cornflour
Flour, plain, wholemeal
Flour, self-raising, wholemeal
Hazelnuts, unsalted, roasted
Hemp seeds
Linseeds
LSA (linseed, sunflower and almond meal)
Macadamias, unsalted
Macaroni
Oat bran
Pasta, wholemeal, any shape
Peanuts, crushed
Pecans
Pine nuts
Pistachios, unsalted
Polenta, fine and instant
Pumpkin seeds
Quinoa
Rice flour
Rice noodles, vermicelli
Rice noodles, wide
Rice, arborio
Rice, basmati
Rice, brown
Rolled oats
Sesame seeds
Spaghetti, wholemeal
Sunflower seeds
Walnuts

Sauces and pastes

Curry paste, red
Curry paste, yellow
Fish sauce
Hoisin sauce
Sambal oelek (chilli paste)
Sweet chilli sauce
Tomato passata
Tomato paste
Worcestershire sauce

Spices, herbs and condiments

Almond butter
Basil, dried
Cayenne pepper
Chilli flakes, dried
Chilli powder
Cinnamon, ground
Coriander, ground
Cumin, ground
Curry powder
Dukkah
Garam masala
Garlic powder
Ginger, ground
Honey
Italian herbs, dried
Maple syrup, pure
Mayonnaise, reduced fat
Molasses, pure
Mustard powder
Mustard, dijon
Mustard, wholegrain
Nutmeg, ground

Onion powder
Oregano, dried
Paprika, smoked
Peanut butter
Pepper, black
Rosemary, dried
Salt
Sauerkraut
Strawberry jam, sugar-free
Tahini
Tamari
Thyme, dried
Turmeric, ground
Vinegar, apple cider
Vinegar, red wine
Vinegar, rice wine
Vinegar, white

Oils

Coconut oil
Cooking oil spray
Extra-virgin olive oil

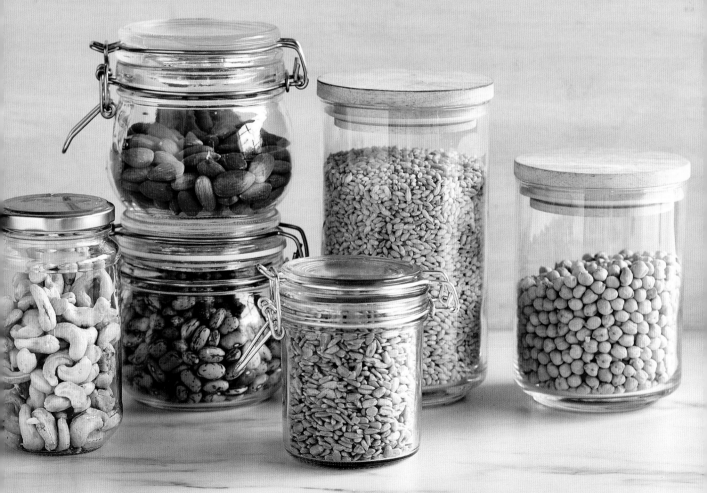

GET COOKING!

You've prepared your meal plan, you've done your budget shopping and now you're ready to put everything into action.

Losing weight and maintaining a healthy lifestyle on a budget is all about preparation, so bulk cooking is one of the key tools to reach your goals.

Choose a day or two each week when you've got some time to do your meal preparation and bulk cooking. It'll keep you in a routine and ensure that you're organised, and not making last-minute (usually unhealthy) food choices.

TOP TIPS FOR MEAL PREP AND BULK COOKING

Double every recipe

Freeze half and use another time or have it for lunch the next day. So many meals are freezer friendly: chilli con carne, curries, pasta sauces, cooked meatballs, rissoles, stews, pasta bakes, pies, casseroles etc. To help with your planning, we clearly indicate which recipes in this book are suitable to freeze.

Peel, chop and grate

This counts as prep, too! Get ingredients ready in advance and store them in airtight containers in the fridge for a great head start when cooking and assembling meals.

Be a portion queen

Choose three or four recipes with similar ingredients and make five or six serves of each. Portion each recipe into containers and freeze or refrigerate, depending on when you're going to eat them.

Multitask

Have something in the oven, in the slow cooker and on the stovetop at the same time to enable you to cook more in one sitting and make the most of your bulk shopping.

Bulk bake snacks

While you're having your bulk-cooking session, choose two or three healthy snacks to make, too. Freezer-friendly items, such as muffins, slices or bliss balls, are great to have on hand and will stop you reaching for an unhealthy option.

Smooth(ie) operator

Package up your favourite smoothie combinations and freeze them in single-portion containers. Then you can just throw the contents in a blender, add milk or yoghurt and blitz for a speedy and healthy snack, breakfast or lunch.

Get the family involved

Encourage the kids to help you peel, slice, grate, stir and prepare dishes. It'll save you time and get everyone interested in the healthy food you're preparing. The same goes for cleaning up; get the kids to help out and they'll learn that healthy eating is something for everyone to participate in.

Your initial motivation to bulk cook and meal prep will get you started. Keep going so it becomes a habit to help you reach your weight-loss goals and choose healthy options most of the time.

Handy hint: The more you schedule in a bulk-cooking session as an enjoyable thing to do, the more likely you are to stick to it and save money by being so organised.

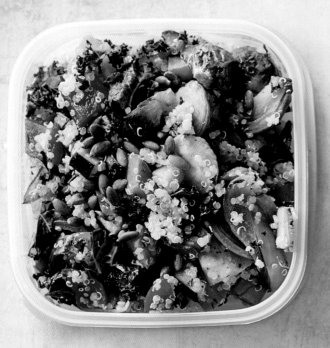
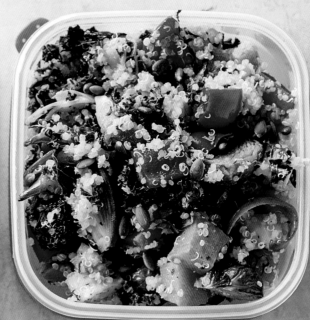
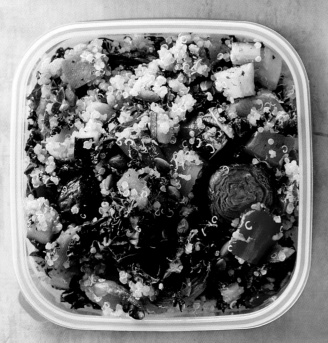
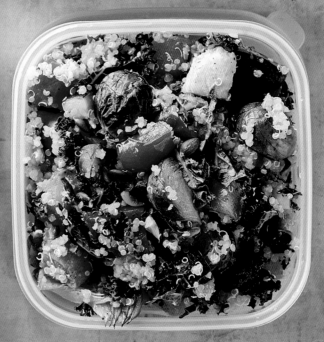

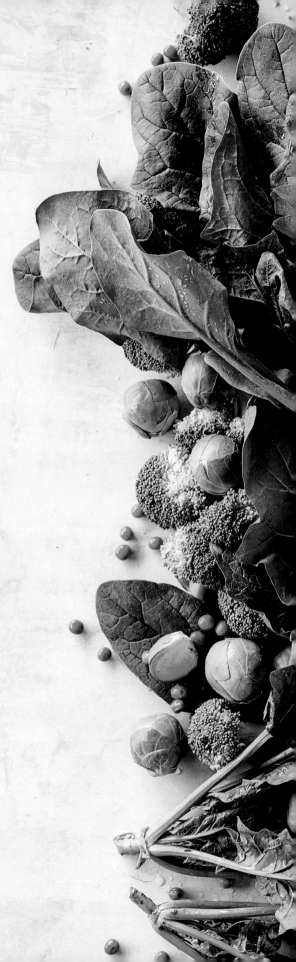

MEAL PREP TOOLS

Meal prep is much easier with the help of some essential tools. Most of the items listed below are inexpensive and, even if they require an upfront outlay, once you have them you'll be able to regularly cook in bulk, which in turn will save you money.

Blender

Whether it's a benchtop option or a stick blender these are great for blitzing up soups, smoothies, desserts, pancake batters and so on.

Clean pots and pans

After each meal-prep session, clean your pots, pans and utensils thoroughly and store for their next use. Having to scrub a load of dishes before you can even think about cooking isn't fun for anyone!

Food processor

It doesn't have to be an expensive one, but they do make dicing and slicing veggies and other ingredients a lot faster than chopping everything by hand.

Kettle

Don't wait for a large pot of water to come to the boil on the stovetop; pre-boil water in the kettle and you'll have pasta, rice and quinoa cooking faster. Also great for soaking noodles for stir-fries and salads.

Kitchen scissors

Use these to cut bacon, spring onions, fresh herbs and other soft ingredients directly into your saucepans or serving dishes.

Mandoline

Slicing vegetables with a mandoline will save you time chopping and, if your veggies are washed well, there's no need to peel them. Thinly sliced veggies take less time to cook, too.

Rice cooker

Cook rice perfectly every time with a simple rice cooker. Having batches of rice prepared in advance to serve with your meals makes things much faster at dinner time. Ensure you store cooked rice safely (see the pull-out fridge poster for storage basics) and always reheat to steaming before serving.

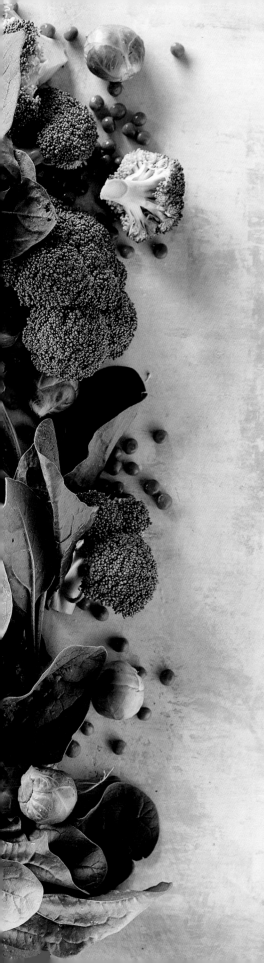

Sharp knives

Ensure the knives you use are always sharp, so you can slice and dice quickly and safely.

Slow cooker

You should be able to pick up a good slow cooker for under $50 and it will make your meal prep so much easier. Place all the ingredients in the cooker in the morning and by the afternoon you'll have a delicious healthy meal, ready to eat or store for another day.

Storage containers

There's no point in preparing loads of meals in bulk if you can't store them easily and effectively in the fridge or freezer. You don't need expensive containers; they just need to stack easily and seal well.

STORE IN BULK

Assess your storage options before you buy groceries in bulk and start making loads of meals. There's no point in preparing more than you can store.

Try some of these tips for storing prepared meals and leftovers, helping you to save money and avoid waste.

- Freeze sauces, curries, stews etc in zip-lock bags. Remove as much air as possible and lay them flat in the freezer. Not only does this save space, it also makes thawing meals super speedy.

- Always label and date the containers you store your prepared meals in, being sure to rotate them if you're adding regularly to your stash.

- Freeze fruit and veggies before they end up in the compost bin. Cut up larger items and place in containers or zip-lock bags. Always peel bananas before freezing.

- When fruit and veggies are on special or in season, you can buy them in bulk and freeze for later, to save money and ensure that you're stocked up with healthy ingredients.

- Leftover staples, such as rice and quinoa, can be stored in an airtight container in the fridge for about 3 days or in the freezer for several months. Remember, food safety is particularly important with high-moisture foods such as these, so only ever reheat them once and be sure they are heated to steaming.

- Throw leftover rice or quinoa into a frittata or soup, serve with a veggie stir-fry or use to make a quick fried rice. You can also have it cold for breakfast as a rustic rice pudding (add milk, a little honey and some fresh fruit), or whip up some sushi for lunch.

- Eat leftover cooked meats for lunch the next day or pop them into a salad or sandwich.

- If you are not a family of bread 'end' lovers, save the ends of your bread in a bag in the freezer and use to make breadcrumbs.

- If you get towards the end of the week and your fresh herbs are looking a little limp, chop them up and place in ice-cube trays with a little stock, water or oil, and you'll have instant flavour cubes to add to your meals.

- Save yourself some money and reuse glass jars rather than buying loads of containers or freezer bags. Glass can be frozen, too – just be sure not to overfill the jar.

Team Tip

'I've gone from stay-at-home mum to working full time, so I pre-make and freeze hidden veg sausage rolls and pies, which we can reheat on nights when we don't have much time. I rotate through a few family favourite meals when we don't get home until 6 pm and everyone's grumpy. Lunches are usually a mixture of leftovers or a salad that has similar ingredients and I can change the dressing so I don't get bored.' – FLIP

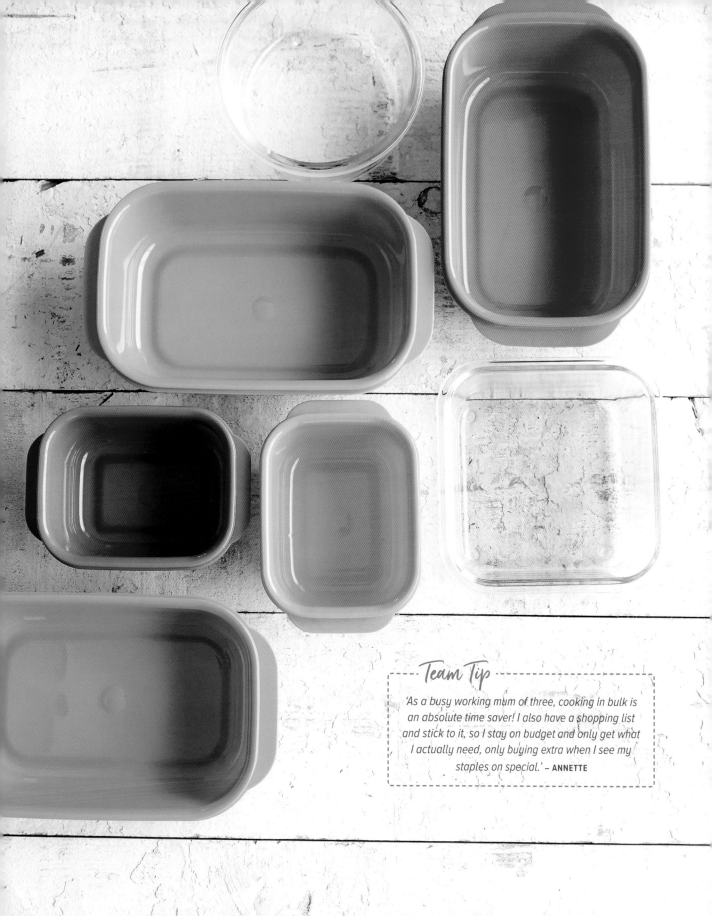

RUN A HEALTHY AND BUDGET-FRIENDLY HOUSEHOLD

You probably already work to a household budget and have an idea of how much you need to spend on essential items, and what's left over for family entertainment and the fun stuff in life.

To lose weight on a budget, there are a few key areas where you can save money and still reach your healthy-lifestyle goals.

EXERCISE MORE

Simply being more active in and around the house is a perfectly good way to lose weight and see results.

Run, don't walk

Start jogging or run around with the kids at the park. There are loads of exercises you can do to lose weight without breaking the bank.

Get out of the house

If you have a dog, even better. Use the dog as your non-negotiable reason to get out every day, even just for a 20-minute walk.

Use an app

Apps (such as The Healthy Mummy app) provide you with video workouts that you can do at home. Go to healthymummy.com to access.

Choose incidental exercise

Try taking the stairs instead of the lift, walking to the shops rather than driving, squatting between hanging each piece of clothing on the washing line, or lunging while you're waiting for the kettle to boil. You can move more all the time – it's free and it's amazing for weight loss!

> *Team Tip*
>
> *'I cook a whole chicken in the slow cooker on a Sunday and use it in all sorts of dishes, such as Asian chicken salad for lunch, chicken sandwiches for the kids or chicken noodle soup. I use the stock for soups and curries so nothing is wasted.'*
> **– ISABELLA**

EATING OUT

Eating out is probably something you want to cut back on anyway while you're trying to lose weight, as restaurant, cafe and pub meals aren't always the healthiest option. On the plus side, it'll save you money! If you *are* eating out, here are some budget-friendly ideas.

Choose a vegetarian option

These are often cheaper than meat-based dishes.

Pick an entree and a side salad

Still a satisfying meal, but cheaper than an entree and a main, and it will stop you overeating.

Skip dessert

Have a healthy snack (if you need it) when you get home.

Order by the glass

If you enjoy an alcoholic drink, try and stick to just one or two glasses.

Share

Choose a larger main meal you can share with a friend or your partner.

Ask for the kids' menu

If the kids are with you, their menu often has smaller meals (avoiding waste) that are lower in price and sometimes come as a 'meal deal', including a drink and dessert.

> *Team Tip*
>
> *'I focus on my "weak" meal type, where I've fallen down in the past. My weak link is snacks, so I make sure I have heaps prepped.'* **– TITANIA**

LUNCHBOXES

Whether you're making lunchboxes for the kids, your partner or yourself, keep them healthy and budget friendly by following these tips.

Snack sensibly

Divide your bulk-bought food among reusable lunchbox containers. A large bag of popcorn makes a healthy morning snack for the whole family and can be divided into individual portions to make it more cost effective. Even better, a piece of fruit, some crackers and cheese or homemade dip are inexpensive and will keep you on track with your weight-loss goals.

Make your own

Choose one or two healthy snacks each week, such as slices, muffins or bliss balls, and prepare them in advance.

Use up leftovers

Save time and money by taking advantage of the office microwave to reheat leftovers for lunch. A thermos is a great option for the kids, as they generally don't have access to a kitchen at school.

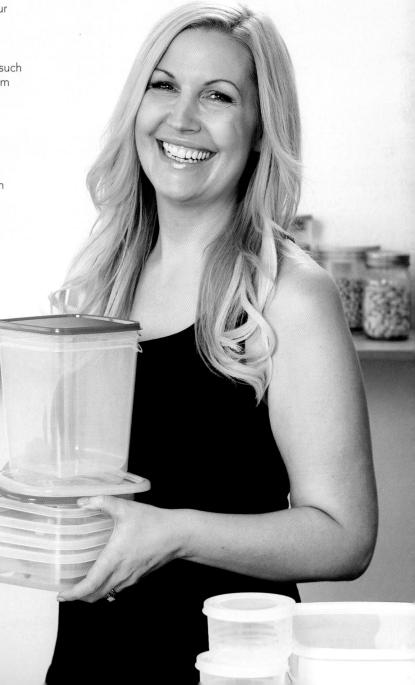

- - - - Team Tip - - - -

'I use hummus for everything – as a delicious protein-packed sauce for pasta or veggies, as a spread instead of cheese or butter, and as a dip for snacks. It saves me when I get home from work and need to make a quick dinner, or when I'm prepping lunchboxes or snacks. I always have a batch ready to go.' – JEN

MEET SOME AMAZING MUMS

Case Study One: *Cicily*, mum of two, Nambucca Heads, NSW

Cicily has been part of The Healthy Mummy community for 18 months and has lost 53 kg.

Before joining The Healthy Mummy, Cicily was not the happy and vivacious mum she is today. In fact, she says she was in denial and would always pretend to be really confident. 'I tried to put on a happy and confident facade, when in fact I was depressed and anxious – without really understanding that I was unhappy in myself. I just blamed the world and everyone else and didn't really put it on me.'

Cicily has now transformed both her and her family's lives. 'I finally feel like I get to be me; the person I've always wanted to be but have always kept hidden. It's like I've opened up a whole new world. This is who I am meant to be and everything seems so much easier.'

Not only have Cicily's health and fitness changed forever, her confidence has soared.

Cicily's top tips

1. TRY SOMETHING NEW
I try all sorts of foods I would never have tried before, things that I wouldn't even think about. I've never had something that I don't like.

2. DAZZLE THE DOUBTERS
There are so many things my partner doesn't eat – eggs, nuts, fish, seafood, mushrooms, anything creamy, anything green. I *still* find recipes to feed him and my family.

3. JOIN THE COMMUNITY
I love getting to know other women who have changed their lives so much. You bond and connect so well, and form beautiful friendships.

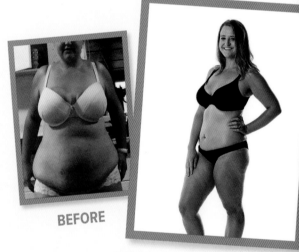

BEFORE

AFTER

Case Study Two: *Elle*, mum of one, Perth, WA

Elle has been part of The Healthy Mummy community for 3 years and has lost 20 kg.

After breaking up with her son's father, Elle turned to binge eating to cope with her emotions.

But even though she ate to try and make herself feel better, she says it had the opposite effect. 'So this time I decided to be strong, power through and not use food as a comfort,' Elle says.

Since losing 20 kg, Elle has been able to run for 21 km and has competed in a power-lifting contest. With another competition approaching, she's aiming to weigh around 60–62 kg, keep her body fat down, and gain strength and muscle. She's well on her way to that goal by walking and playing with her son, and training four times a week.

Elle has not only overhauled her fitness, she's also changed her eating and shopping habits. 'I definitely buy less packaged food and I buy things like chicken and beef in bulk, always free-range and as fresh as possible. I remind myself that my journey is for my health and energy, and not just for weight loss.'

Elle's power prompts

1. PREPARE TO PREP
Make brekkie the night before to stop yourself from choosing bad options and/or overeating.

2. BULK IT UP
Meal prep once or twice a week by choosing meals, cooking them in bulk and then storing or freezing them.

3. CONSISTENCY IS KEY
Be consistent, but don't worry too much if you slip up – it happens!

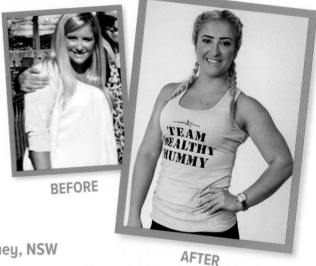

BEFORE

AFTER

Case Study Three: *Melissa*, mum of two, Sydney, NSW

Melissa has been part of The Healthy Mummy community for 6 months and has lost 32 kg.

After losing 32 kg on The Healthy Mummy program, Melissa already loves her body. But she's determined to reach her final goal and boost her confidence in the process. 'By the end of this year I want to be 100 per cent confident with my body and be able to fit into a size 8. I'm currently a 10,' she says.

Melissa is now down to 73 kg and is looking forward to getting to 70 kg by building and toning her muscles.

Melissa's food fixes

1. SHAKE IT UP
Try a smoothie for breakfast or lunch. Include protein and fruit to ensure it's filling and full of deliciously healthy ingredients.

2. PACK IN PROTEIN
Keep protein levels high to stay fuller for longer.

3. START SMART SNACKING
Hummus and fruit are my picks for snacks on the go.

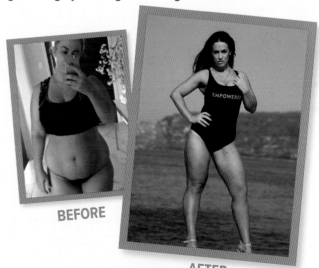

BEFORE

AFTER

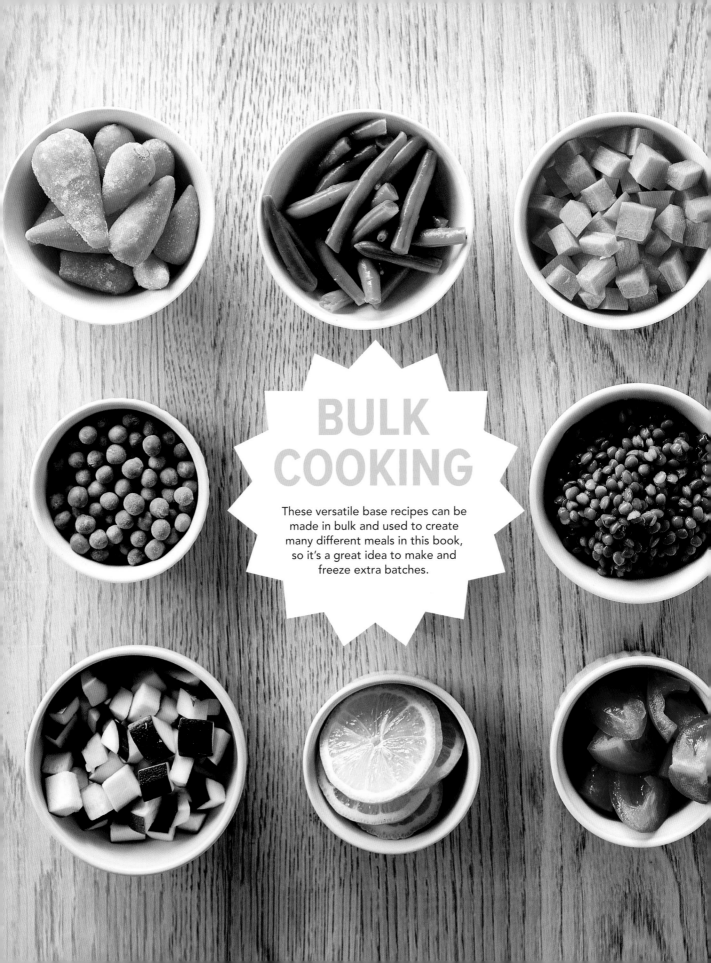

BULK COOKING

These versatile base recipes can be made in bulk and used to create many different meals in this book, so it's a great idea to make and freeze extra batches.

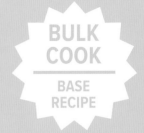

ROASTED RAINBOW VEGGIES

Double or triple this base recipe to make the following meals:

- *Roasted Rainbow Veggie Breakfast Salad (p. 80)*
- *Roasted Rainbow Veggie, Kale and Quinoa Salad (p. 100)*
- *Spiced Chicken and Roasted Rainbow Veggie Tacos (p. 191)*

SERVES
4

PREPARATION
15 MINS

COOK
45 MINS (4 HOURS IN A SLOW COOKER)

COST PER SERVE
$1.71

240 g pumpkin, peeled and seeds removed, diced
240 g sweet potato, peeled and diced
2 red capsicums, diced
2 small zucchini, diced
2 small red onions, cut into wedges
200 g brussels sprouts, trimmed and halved
2 parsnips, peeled and diced
2 tablespoons extra-virgin olive oil
2 teaspoons dried Italian herbs
salt and freshly ground black pepper

Place all the vegetables in a large bowl with the olive oil and dried herbs. Season with salt and pepper and toss well to combine.

If cooking in the oven:
Preheat the oven to 200°C and line a baking tray with baking paper.

Spread the mixed veggies over the tray in a single layer and roast for 30–45 minutes until golden and tender.

If cooking in a slow cooker:
Place the veggies in the slow cooker dish and cook on high, stirring frequently, for 2–4 hours until tender.

Store leftover roasted rainbow veggies in an airtight container in the fridge for 3–4 days or freeze for up to 3 months.

SUITABLE TO FREEZE

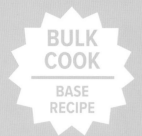

PULLED PORK

Double or triple this base recipe to make the following meals:

- *Zesty Greek Salad with Pulled Pork (p. 110)*
- *Pulled Pork, Rice and Kale Salad (p. 111)*
- *Pulled Pork and Spinach Sloppy Joes (p. 163)*

SERVES
6

PREPARATION
15 MINS

COOK
3 HOURS (8 HOURS IN A SLOW COOKER)

COST PER SERVE
$0.73

2 teaspoons smoked paprika
½ teaspoon chilli powder
½ teaspoon garlic powder
¼ teaspoon dried thyme
2 teaspoons honey
1 tablespoon red wine vinegar
1 teaspoon pure molasses
500 g boneless pork shoulder, trimmed
salt and freshly ground black pepper
1 teaspoon extra-virgin olive oil
½ brown onion, finely sliced

Combine the paprika, chilli powder, garlic powder, thyme, honey, vinegar and molasses in a bowl to form a paste. Rub the paste all over the pork, season with salt and pepper and set aside.

Heat the olive oil in a flameproof casserole dish over medium–high heat and cook the onion for 1–2 minutes until translucent. If you are cooking the pork in a slow cooker, the onion can be cooked in a saucepan or frying pan, then transferred to the slow cooker dish.

If cooking on the stovetop:
Place the pork on top of the onion in the casserole dish and pour over ½ cup of water. Cover the dish with a lid, reduce the heat to low and simmer for 2½–3 hours, rotating the pork regularly, until the meat is very tender. Add a little extra water if the pork starts to dry out at any point. Remove the pork from the dish and set aside.

Pour the cooking liquid into a bowl and allow to cool, skimming off the fat as it rises. Once the fat has been removed, return the liquid to the casserole dish. Bring to the boil, then reduce the heat and simmer for a few minutes until thickened slightly.

Using two forks, shred the pork into small pieces. Add the shredded pork to the thickened sauce and stir to combine.

If cooking in a slow cooker:
Place the pork, onion and ½ cup of water in the slow cooker dish and cook on low for 8 hours until the meat is very tender. Remove the pork from the cooker and set aside.

Pour the cooking liquid into a bowl and allow to cool, skimming off the fat as it rises. Once the fat has been removed, pour the liquid into a saucepan. Bring to the boil, then reduce the heat and simmer for a few minutes until thickened slightly.

Using two forks, shred the pork into small pieces. Add the shredded pork to the thickened sauce and stir to combine.

Store leftover pulled pork in an airtight container in the fridge for 3–4 days or freeze for up to 3 months.

SUITABLE TO FREEZE

CAJUN CHICKEN

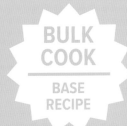

BULK COOK

BASE RECIPE

Double or triple this base recipe to make the following meals:

- *Cajun Chicken Salad Bowl (p. 114)*
- *Cajun Chicken Pizzas (p. 189)*
- *Cajun Chicken Meatballs (p. 215)*

SERVES
6

PREPARATION
10 MINS

COOK
1 HOUR (3 HOURS IN A SLOW COOKER)

COST PER SERVE
$0.91

1 teaspoon ground cumin
1 teaspoon ground coriander
1 teaspoon smoked paprika
¾ teaspoon dried oregano
¾ teaspoon dried basil
¾ teaspoon dried thyme
1½ teaspoons cayenne
   pepper
500 g chicken breast fillets
salt and freshly ground
   black pepper
1 cup salt-reduced chicken
   stock, plus extra if needed

Combine all the spices and dried herbs in a bowl. Add the chicken and thoroughly coat in the spice mix. Season well with salt and pepper.

If cooking in the oven:
Preheat the oven to 180°C.

Place the spiced chicken in a casserole dish and pour over the stock. Cover with a lid and bake for 1 hour until the chicken is very tender. Add some extra stock or water during cooking if the chicken starts to dry out.

Using two forks, shred the chicken into bite-sized pieces.

If cooking in a slow cooker:
Place the spiced chicken and chicken stock in the slow cooker dish. Cover with the lid and cook on medium for 3 hours. Add some extra stock or water during cooking if the chicken starts to dry out.

Using two forks, shred the chicken into bite-sized pieces.

Store leftover Cajun chicken in an airtight container in the fridge for 3–4 days or freeze for up to 2 months.

SUITABLE TO FREEZE

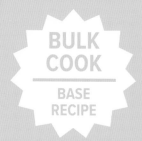

HIDDEN VEG BOLOGNESE

Double or triple this base recipe to make the following meals:

- *Zoodles with Hidden Veg Bolognese (p. 144)*
- *Hidden Veg Bolognese Pie (p. 196)*
- *Hidden Veg Bolognese Potatoes (p. 197)*

SERVES
4

PREPARATION
10 MINS

COOK
50 MINS

COST PER SERVE
$1.18

1 tablespoon extra-virgin olive oil
2 garlic cloves, grated
160 g lean beef mince
160 g lean pork mince
1 carrot, diced
120 g pumpkin, peeled and seeds removed, diced
1 celery stalk, diced
½ red capsicum, diced
200 g canned diced tomatoes
1 tablespoon tomato paste
1 cup salt-reduced beef stock
½ teaspoon dried Italian herbs
salt and freshly ground black pepper

FOR A VEGETARIAN MEAL

Use vegetable stock and replace the mince with 2 × 400 g cans of lentils, drained and rinsed.

Heat the olive oil in a large heavy-based saucepan over medium–high heat. Add the garlic and beef and pork mince and cook, breaking up any lumps with the back of a wooden spoon, for 4–5 minutes until the meat is browned all over.

Stir in the carrot, pumpkin, celery and capsicum and cook for 1–2 minutes. Add the canned tomatoes, tomato paste and stock. Bring to the boil, then reduce the heat to very low and simmer for 30–40 minutes until the sauce is rich and thickened. Add the dried herbs just before serving and season to taste with salt and pepper.

Store leftover bolognese in an airtight container in the fridge for 2–3 days or freeze for up to 3 months.

SUITABLE TO FREEZE

LAMB AND LENTIL CURRY

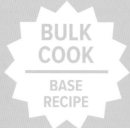

Double or triple this base recipe to make the following meals:

- *Lamb and Lentil Curry with Coriander Rice (p. 171)*
- *Lamb and Lentil Curry-stuffed Zucchini (p. 194)*
- *Lamb and Lentil Curry Pasties (p. 199)*

SERVES
4

PREPARATION
15 MINS

COOK
1 HOUR 50 MINS (6–8 HOURS IN A SLOW COOKER)

COST PER SERVE
$2.20

---

1 tablespoon extra-virgin olive oil
1 brown onion, diced
3 garlic cloves, chopped
340 g boneless lamb shoulder, trimmed and cut into 2 cm cubes
1 tablespoon curry powder
2 tablespoons garam masala
½ teaspoon ground turmeric
freshly ground black pepper
1 × 400 g can brown lentils, drained and rinsed
1 × 400 g can chopped tomatoes
1 cup salt-reduced chicken stock
1 potato, diced
1 carrot, diced
1 small zucchini, diced
120 g green beans, trimmed and halved

FOR A VEGETARIAN MEAL

Omit the lamb, use vegetable stock and add 320 g diced sweet potato and a drained 400 g can of corn kernels to the curry.

Heat the olive oil in a deep heavy-based saucepan or flameproof casserole dish over medium–high heat, add the onion and garlic and cook for 1–2 minutes until the onion is translucent.

Add the lamb and cook for 3–4 minutes until browned all over. Now add the curry powder, garam masala, turmeric and a good pinch of pepper and stir to combine.

If cooking on the stovetop:
Add the lentils, canned tomatoes and stock and mix well. Cover and cook over medium–low heat for 1¼ hours. Add the potato and carrot and cook for a further 15–20 minutes until the lamb is tender. Finally, add the zucchini and beans and cook for a further 10 minutes until all the vegetables are cooked through.

If cooking in a slow cooker:
Transfer the lamb mixture to the slow cooker dish. Mix in the lentils, canned tomatoes, stock, potato, carrot, zucchini, beans and 1 cup of water. Cover and cook on low heat for 6–8 hours or high heat for 3–4 hours. Add more water if the sauce starts to dry out.

Store leftover curry in an airtight container in the fridge for 4–5 days or freeze for up to 3 months.

SUITABLE TO FREEZE

BREAKFAST

Start the day right!

OVEN-BAKED MAPLE AND BANANA FRENCH TOAST

SERVES
6

PREPARATION
10 MINS

COOK
45 MINS

COST PER SERVE
$1.41

cooking oil spray (optional)
6 slices wholegrain or gluten-free bread of choice
6 free-range eggs
2 ¼ cups unsweetened almond milk
1 teaspoon ground cinnamon
1 tablespoon vanilla extract
2 tablespoons pure maple syrup
pinch of salt
4 small bananas, sliced
1 tablespoon coconut sugar
20 g unsalted butter
1 tablespoon cacao nibs

NUTRI DETAILS PER SERVE

1398 kJ/333 cals	Sat fat: 3.8 g
Protein: 12.9 g	Carbs: 41.1 g
Fibre: 4.8 g	Total sugar: 18.7 g
Total fat: 12.2 g	Free sugar: 7.2 g

Preheat the oven to 180°C. Line a large baking dish with baking paper or lightly spray with cooking oil.

Arrange the bread slices over the base of the prepared dish (it's fine if they overlap slightly).

Place the eggs, milk, cinnamon, vanilla, maple syrup and salt in a bowl and whisk for 1–2 minutes until smooth and well combined. Pour the mixture over the bread slices in the dish to saturate the bread. Bake for 45 minutes until golden and the custard is set.

About 15 minutes before the French toast is ready, combine the banana slices with the sugar.

Melt the butter in a medium frying pan over medium heat. Add the banana slices and cook for 2 minutes on each side until the banana is lightly golden and caramelised.

Serve one piece of French toast per person with some of the caramelised banana and a sprinkle of cacao nibs.

Store any leftovers in an airtight container in the fridge for 3–4 days.

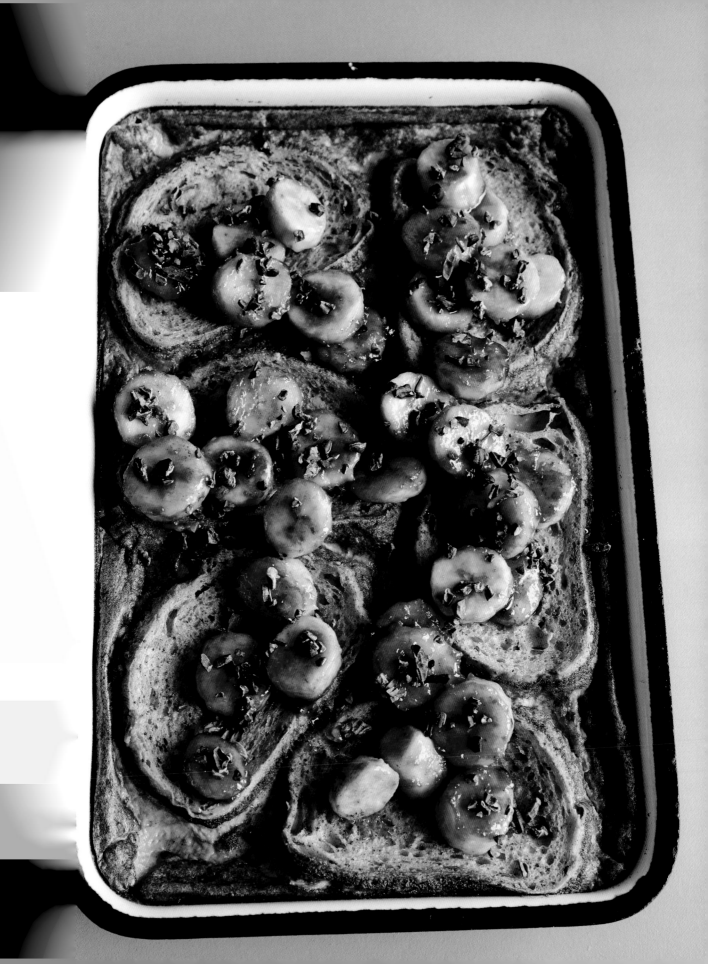

APPLE AND BLUEBERRY CORNBREAD

SERVES
6

PREPARATION
5 MINS

COOK
30 MINS

COST PER SERVE
$1.33

2 cups instant polenta
1 cup cornflour
2 teaspoons baking powder
1 small apple, grated
1 tablespoon stevia powder
1 cup blueberries
    (fresh or frozen)
1 free-range egg,
    lightly beaten
2 cups reduced-fat milk
    of choice
1 teaspoon coconut oil
½ cup reduced-fat plain
    Greek yoghurt
1½ tablespoons honey

NUTRI DETAILS PER SERVE

1405 kJ/334 cals	Sat fat: 1.5 g
Protein: 9.2 g	Carbs: 63.6 g
Fibre: 2.4 g	Total sugar: 15 g
Total fat: 4.2 g	Free sugar: 2.9 g

Preheat the oven to 180°C.

Combine the polenta, cornflour, baking powder, grated apple, stevia and blueberries in a bowl. Stir through the egg and milk until combined.

Melt the coconut oil in an ovenproof chargrill pan or cast-iron frying pan over medium heat. Pour in the batter and cook for 2–3 minutes until just starting to set.

Transfer the pan to the oven and cook for a further 20–25 minutes until the cornbread is cooked through and set. (Start checking after 20 minutes as you don't want to overcook it.) Cracks will appear on the surface when it's ready; as soon as you see these, remove the cornbread from the oven so it remains fluffy.

Cut into six even slices. Serve one slice per person dolloped with a tablespoon of yoghurt and a teaspoon of honey.

Cover and store any leftovers in the fridge for 4–5 days or wrap individual slices and freeze for up to 2 months.

SUITABLE TO FREEZE

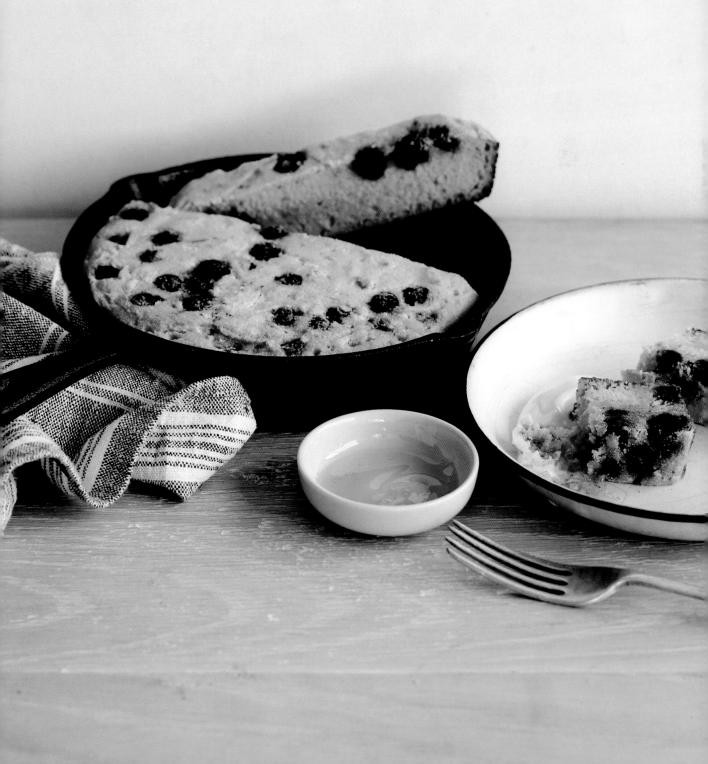

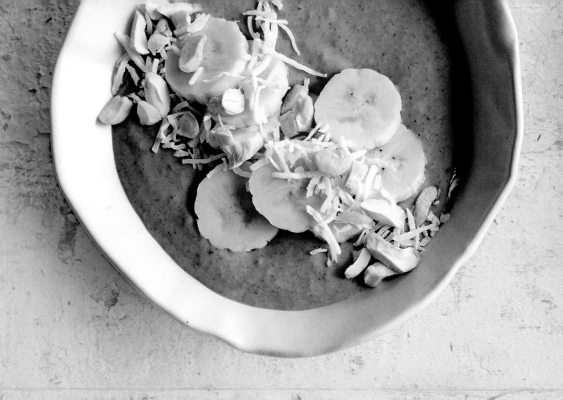

CHOC–BANANA BREAKFAST BOWL

SERVES
1

PREPARATION
5 MINS

COST PER SERVE
$1.55

¾ cup reduced-fat plain
  Greek yoghurt
½ teaspoon stevia powder
2 teaspoons cacao powder
1 small banana
2 teaspoons shredded
  coconut
2 teaspoons unsalted
  cashews, chopped

Place the yoghurt, stevia , cacao powder and half the banana in a blender and blitz until smooth. Scoop into a bowl.

Slice the remaining banana and arrange over the top. Sprinkle over the shredded coconut and cashews and serve.

NUTRI DETAILS PER SERVE

1226 kJ/292 cals	Sat fat: 4.5 g
Protein: 12.9 g	Carbs: 40.6 g
Fibre: 3.3 g	Total sugar: 33.8 g
Total fat: 7.4 g	Free sugar: 0 g

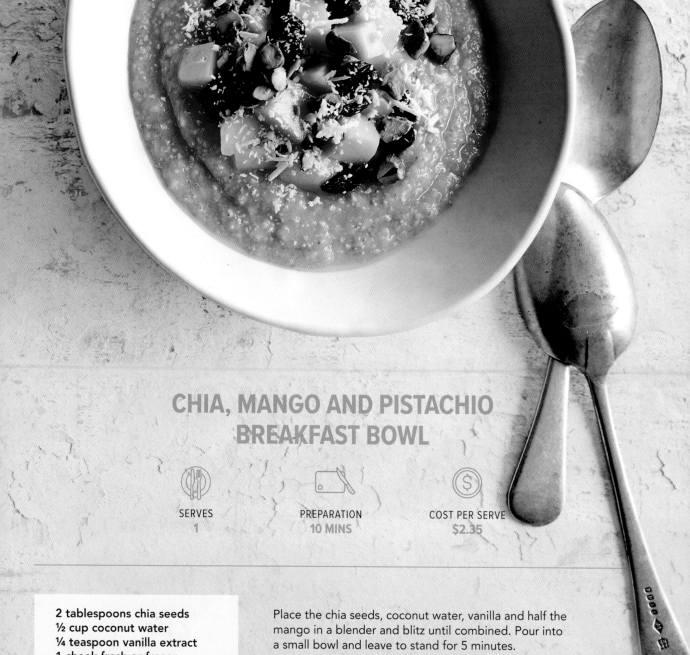

CHIA, MANGO AND PISTACHIO BREAKFAST BOWL

SERVES
1

PREPARATION
10 MINS

COST PER SERVE
$2.35

2 tablespoons chia seeds
½ cup coconut water
¼ teaspoon vanilla extract
1 cheek fresh or frozen mango
1 teaspoon chopped unsalted pistachio kernels
1 teaspoon desiccated coconut
1 teaspoon dried cranberries

Place the chia seeds, coconut water, vanilla and half the mango in a blender and blitz until combined. Pour into a small bowl and leave to stand for 5 minutes.

Chop the remaining mango and scatter it over the chia mixture, along with the pistachios, coconut and cranberries. Serve.

NUTRI DETAILS PER SERVE

1405 kJ/335 cals	Sat fat: 2.3 g
Protein: 8.8 g	Carbs: 46.7 g
Fibre: 13.8 g	Total sugar: 32 g
Total fat: 13 g	Free sugar: 0 g

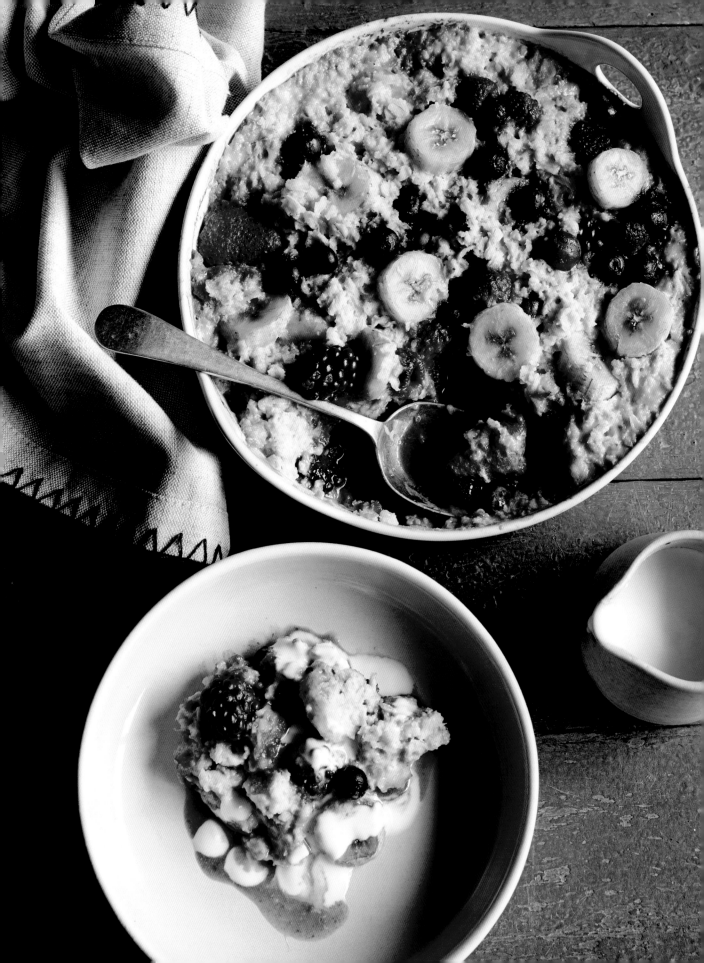

BAKED OATS WITH BANANA AND BERRIES

SERVES
4

PREPARATION
10 MINS

COOK
2 HOURS

COST PER SERVE
$1.05

cooking oil spray
2 cups mixed berries
  (fresh or frozen)
2 small bananas, sliced
1 cup rolled oats
1 cup reduced-fat coconut
  milk, plus extra if needed
1 tablespoon honey

NUTRI DETAILS PER SERVE

1466 kJ/349 cals	Sat fat: 15.3 g
Protein: 6.3 g	Carbs: 36 g
Fibre: 6 g	Total sugar: 19.9 g
Total fat: 19.2 g	Free sugar: 5 g

Preheat the oven to 100°C and lightly spray a medium baking dish with cooking oil.

Layer the berries and sliced banana over the base of the prepared dish. Combine the oats, coconut milk and 1 cup of water in a bowl and pour evenly over the fruit.

Cover the dish with foil and bake for 2 hours until the oats are very tender and all the liquid has been absorbed.

Spoon the baked oats into four bowls. Top each serve with a teaspoon of honey and a little extra coconut milk to loosen the oats if required.

If you're not serving the oats immediately, let them cool, then cover and store in the fridge for up to 3 days. Gently reheat in the oven or microwave before serving.

To save time in the morning, bake the oats in advance, then reheat them when you're ready to serve.

PEANUT BUTTER GRANOLA

SERVES
4

PREPARATION
5 MINS, PLUS
COOLING TIME

COOK
10 MINS

COST PER SERVE
$0.68

⅓ cup peanut butter
2 tablespoons honey
1⅓ cups rolled oats
1 teaspoon ground cinnamon
⅔ cup reduced-fat plain
   Greek yoghurt
⅓ cup blueberries
   (fresh or frozen)

NUTRI DETAILS PER SERVE

1279 kJ/304 cals	Sat fat: 2.3 g
Protein: 10.1 g	Carbs: 37.9 g
Fibre: 4.2 g	Total sugar: 17.2 g
Total fat: 11.7 g	Free sugar: 11 g

Preheat the oven to 180°C. Line a baking tray with baking paper.

Combine the peanut butter and honey in a bowl and microwave in 10-second bursts until the peanut butter has softened. Stir to combine well. Add the oats and stir until the oats are completely coated in the peanut butter mixture.

Spread the mixture over the prepared baking tray and sprinkle with cinnamon. Bake for 8 minutes until the granola is lightly browned. Remove and set aside. It will become crunchy as it cools.

Serve the granola topped with yoghurt and blueberries.

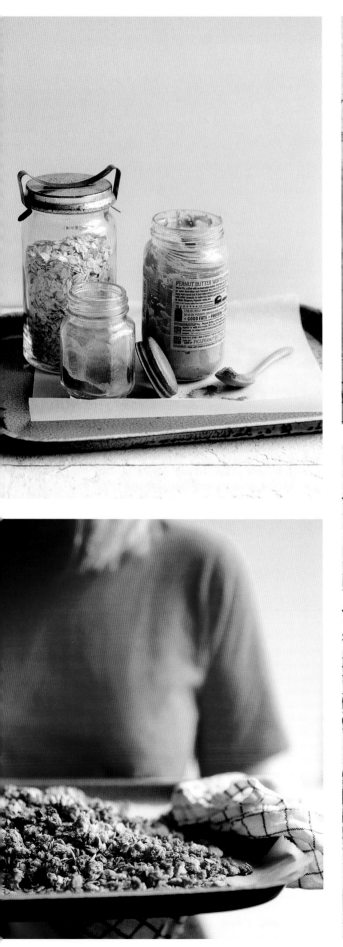
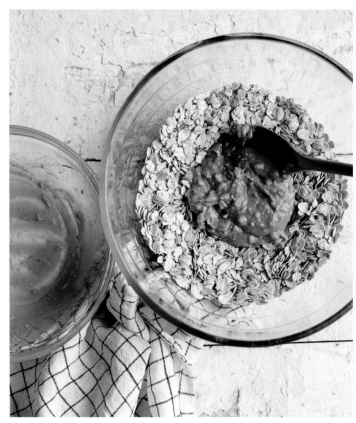
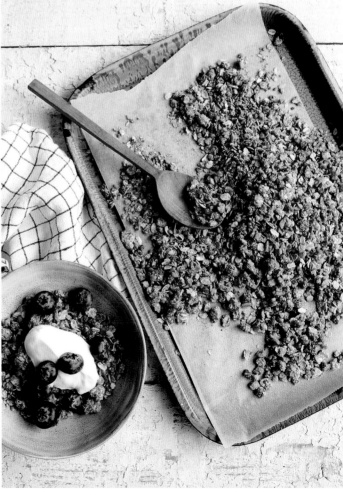

GINGERBREAD PANCAKES

SERVES
4

PREPARATION
5 MINS

COOK
15 MINS

COST PER SERVE
$1.68

1½ cups wholemeal
   self-raising flour
1 teaspoon ground ginger
1 teaspoon ground cinnamon
2 free-range eggs
¾ cup reduced-fat milk
   of choice
40 g butter, melted
½ cup pure maple syrup
1 tablespoon olive oil
1 small banana, sliced

NUTRI DETAILS PER SERVE

1719 kJ/410 cals	Sat fat: 6.9 g
Protein: 9.7 g	Carbs: 55 g
Fibre: 5.8 g	Total sugar: 25 g
Total fat: 15 g	Free sugar: 18 g

In a bowl, stir together the flour, ginger and cinnamon. Set aside.

Lightly beat the eggs and milk in another bowl, then stir in the melted butter and half of the maple syrup. Add the flour mixture and gently fold in until just combined.

Heat a non-stick frying pan over medium heat, drizzle with some of the olive oil and pour ¼ cup of batter for each pancake into the pan. Cook for 2–3 minutes until bubbles appear on the surface, then flip and cook on the other side until golden. Transfer the pancakes to a plate, cover to keep warm, then continue with the remaining olive oil and batter until you have eight pancakes.

Divide the pancakes evenly among four plates. Top with slices of banana, drizzle over the remaining maple syrup and serve.

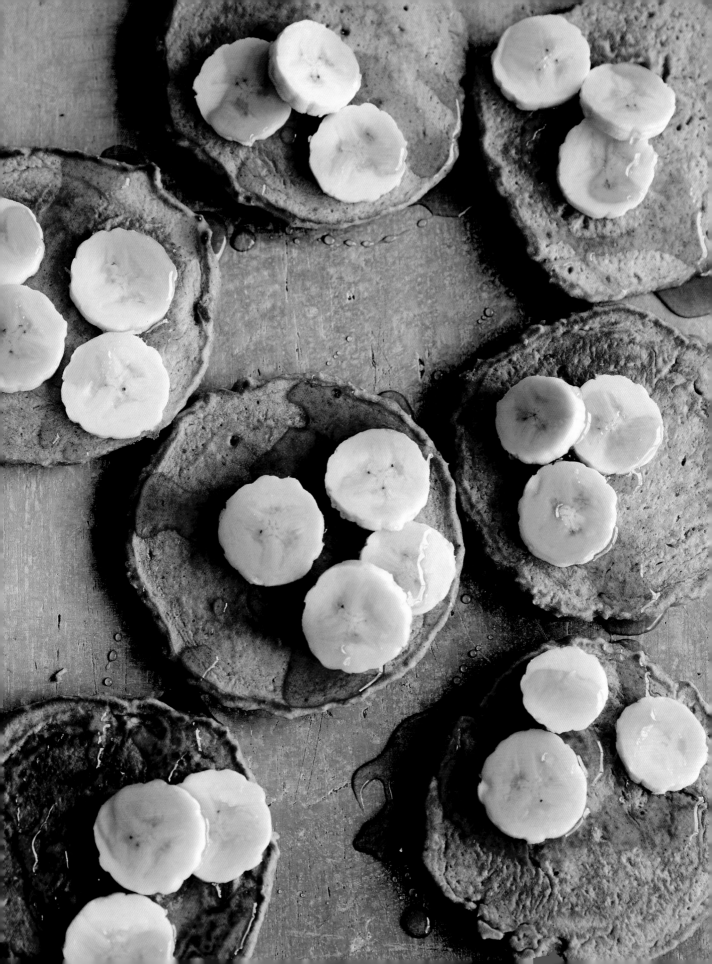

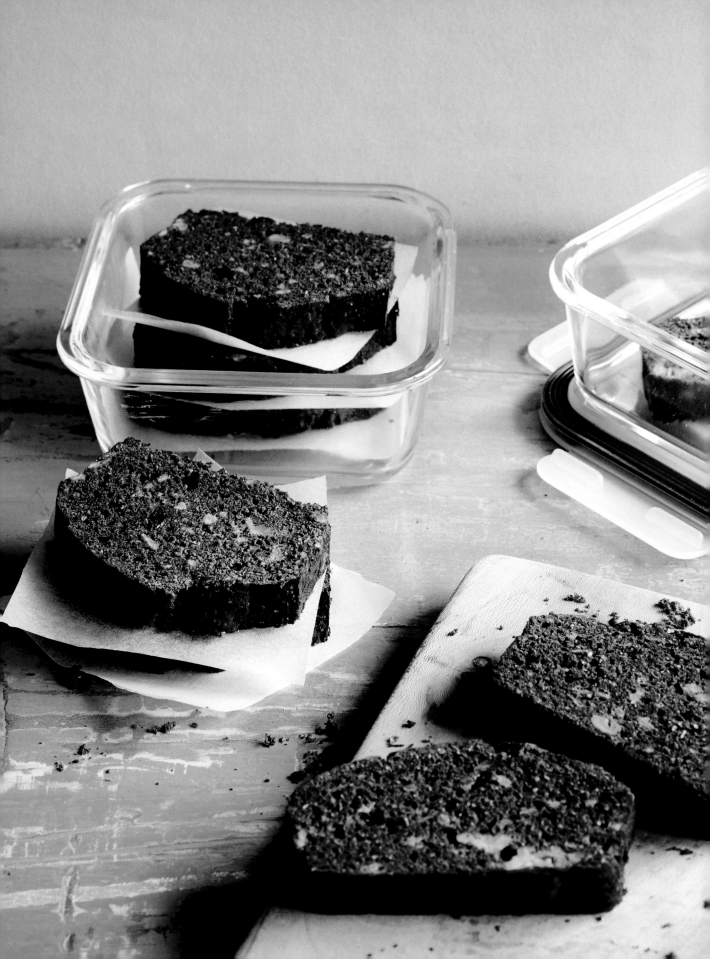

MOCHA BANANA BREAD

SERVES
4

PREPARATION
15 MINS, PLUS
COOLING TIME

COOK
40 MINS

COST PER SERVE
$1.18

cooking oil spray
¾ cup wholemeal plain flour
¼ cup cacao powder
pinch of salt
1 teaspoon baking powder
1 tablespoon chia seeds
½ cup coconut sugar
3 small ripe bananas
2 tablespoons coconut oil, melted
2 free-range eggs
1½ tablespoons pre-made instant coffee

NUTRI DETAILS PER SERVE

1356 kJ/323 cals	Sat fat: 3.8 g
Protein: 9.3 g	Carbs: 54 g
Fibre: 3.9 g	Total sugar: 30.3 g
Total fat: 7 g	Free sugar: 17 g

Preheat the oven to 180°C. Grease and line a standard loaf tin with baking paper.

Combine the flour, cacao powder, salt, baking powder, chia seeds and sugar in a large bowl.

Place the bananas, coconut oil, eggs and coffee in a blender and blitz until well combined but still a bit lumpy.

Fold the banana puree into the flour mixture, then pour the batter into the prepared tin.

Bake for 40 minutes or until a skewer inserted in the centre of the bread comes out clean. Allow to cool in the tin for 5 minutes, then turn out onto a wire rack to cool completely.

Cut the cooled banana bread into eight slices. Two slices is one serve.

Store any leftovers in an airtight container in the fridge for 4–5 days or freeze individual slices for up to 2 months and thaw as required. Try toasting them under the grill to reheat.

SUITABLE TO FREEZE

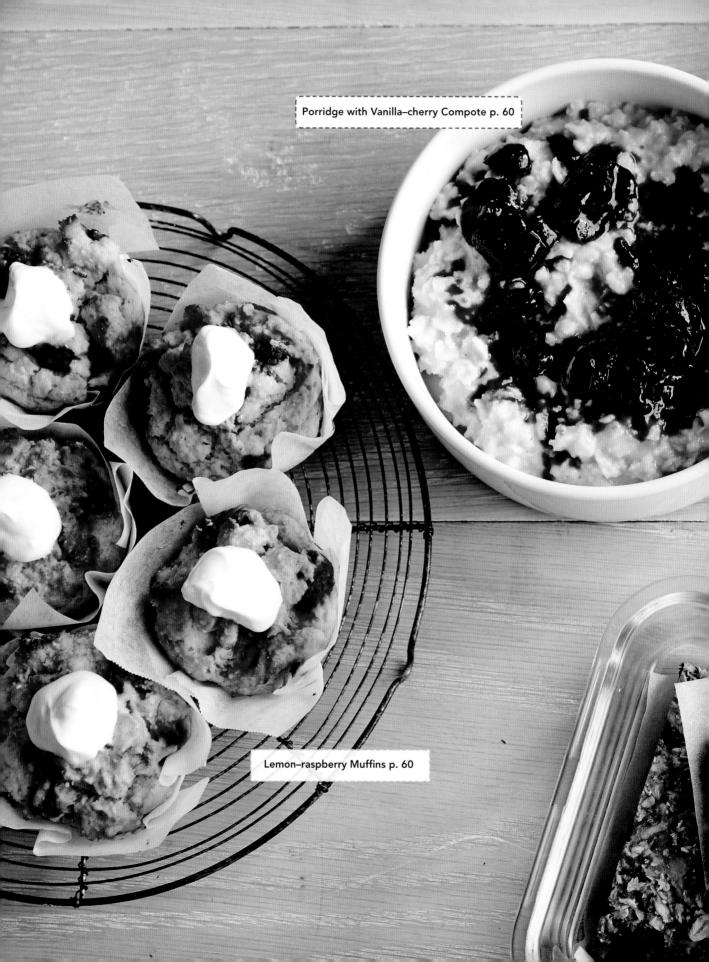

Porridge with Vanilla–cherry Compote p. 60

Lemon–raspberry Muffins p. 60

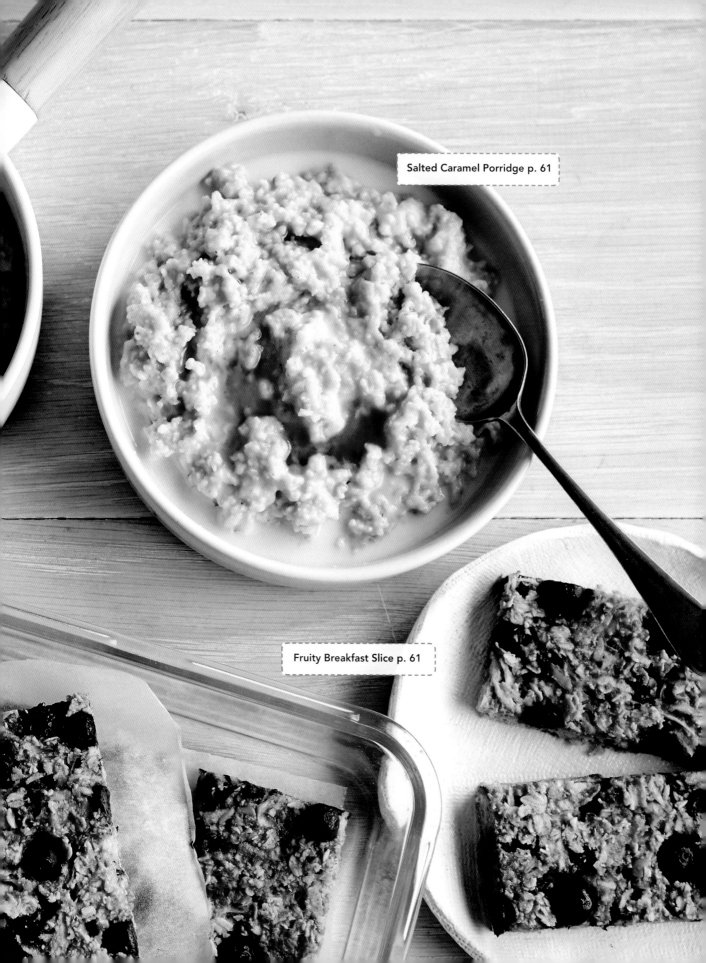

Salted Caramel Porridge p. 61

Fruity Breakfast Slice p. 61

PORRIDGE WITH VANILLA–CHERRY COMPOTE

SERVES	PREPARATION	COOK	COST PER SERVE
1	10 MINS	10 MINS	$1.57

1 cup frozen pitted cherries, chopped
½ teaspoon vanilla extract
1½ tablespoons fresh orange juice
½ cup rolled oats
½ cup reduced-fat milk of choice

Place the cherries, vanilla and orange juice in a small saucepan. Bring to the boil, then reduce the heat and simmer for 5–7 minutes until slightly thickened.

Meanwhile, combine the oats, milk and ½ cup of water in another saucepan and cook, stirring, for 5 minutes until thick and creamy. Thin with a little extra water, if you wish.

Serve the oats with the compote on top.

NUTRI DETAILS PER SERVE

1422 kJ/341 cals	Sat fat: 1.9 g
Protein: 11.8 g	Carbs: 56.8 g
Fibre: 5.9 g	Total sugar: 25.1 g
Total fat: 6.2 g	Free sugar: 2.4 g

LEMON–RASPBERRY MUFFINS

SERVES	PREPARATION	COOK	COST PER SERVE
6	10 MINS, PLUS COOLING TIME	30 MINS	$0.63

cooking oil spray (optional)
1 tablespoon finely grated lemon zest
1 tablespoon lemon juice
1 tablespoon extra-virgin olive oil
¾ cup reduced-fat plain Greek yoghurt
1 cup wholemeal plain flour
1 teaspoon baking powder
¼ cup stevia powder, plus ½ teaspoon extra
½ cup raspberries (fresh or frozen)
¼ cup light cream cheese

Preheat the oven to 180°C. Line or lightly grease six holes of a standard muffin tin.

Combine the lemon zest, lemon juice, olive oil and ⅔ cup of the yoghurt in a bowl.

Mix together the flour, baking powder, ¼ cup of stevia and raspberries in a separate bowl.

Gently fold the yoghurt mixture into the flour mixture until just combined. Divide the batter evenly among the prepared muffin holes.

Bake for 25–30 minutes or until golden and a skewer inserted in the centre of a muffin comes out clean. Cool in the tin for about 5 minutes, then turn out onto a wire rack to cool completely.

Meanwhile, combine the remaining yoghurt, the cream cheese and the extra stevia in a small bowl to make an icing. Dollop a little over each cooled muffin. One muffin is one serve.

Store leftovers in an airtight container in the fridge for 3–4 days or freeze (without icing) for up to 2 months.

SUITABLE TO FREEZE

NUTRI DETAILS PER SERVE

646 kJ/153 cals	Sat fat: 1.9 g
Protein: 5.3 g	Carbs: 17.7 g
Fibre: 3.2 g	Total sugar: 3.3 g
Total fat: 5.7 g	Free sugar: 0 g

FRUITY BREAKFAST SLICE

SERVES
4

PREPARATION
5 MINS

COOK
25 MINS

COST PER SERVE
$1.46

2 cups rolled oats
2 small ripe bananas, mashed
2 granny smith apples, grated
1 cup blueberries (fresh or frozen)
2 free-range eggs, lightly beaten
1 tablespoon LSA (linseed, sunflower
    and almond meal)

Preheat the oven to 180°C and line a 20 cm x 30 cm slice tin with baking paper.

Place all the ingredients in a bowl and mix until well combined. Press the mixture evenly into the prepared tin.

Bake for 20–25 minutes until the slice is golden and firm to the touch. Remove and cool slightly, then cut into 12 even slices. Serve three slices per person.

Store any leftovers in an airtight container in the fridge for 1–2 days or freeze for up to 2 months.

Tip

You could serve this with a dollop of yoghurt, if you like.

SUITABLE TO FREEZE

NUTRI DETAILS PER SERVE

1410 kJ/337 cals	Sat fat: 1.5 g
Protein: 11.6 g	Carbs: 48.5 g
Fibre: 9 g	Total sugar: 18 g
Total fat: 8.5 g	Free sugar: 0 g

SALTED CARAMEL PORRIDGE

SERVES
1

PREPARATION
5 MINS

COOK
5 MINS

COST PER SERVE
$1.46

½ cup rolled oats
100 ml reduced-fat coconut milk
¼ teaspoon vanilla extract
1 teaspoon almond butter
1 teaspoon lemon juice
pinch of salt
1 teaspoon pure maple syrup

Place the oats, coconut milk (reserving some to serve), vanilla, almond butter, lemon juice, salt and 150 ml of water in a saucepan over medium–high heat.

Cook, stirring, for 3–5 minutes until the oats are creamy. Serve immediately with the reserved coconut milk and maple syrup drizzled over the top.

NUTRI DETAILS PER SERVE

1462 kJ/348 cals	Sat fat: 10.9 g
Protein: 7.8 g	Carbs: 38 g
Fibre: 4 g	Total sugar: 5.9 g
Total fat: 17.4 g	Free sugar: 4 g

BREAKFAST TRAY BAKE

SERVES
4

PREPARATION
10 MINS

COOK
1 HOUR (8 HOURS IN
A SLOW COOKER)

COST PER SERVE
$2.11

---

350 g chipolata sausages
2 small sweet potatoes,
    peeled and diced
1 cup salt-reduced
    vegetable stock
2 flat mushrooms,
    finely sliced
1 × 400 g can diced tomatoes
1 tablespoon Worcestershire
    sauce
½ teaspoon smoked paprika
1 garlic clove, crushed
salt and freshly ground
    black pepper
30 g baby spinach leaves
4 slices wholegrain or gluten-
    free bread of choice

NUTRI DETAILS PER SERVE

1309 kJ/313 cals	Sat fat: 3.8 g
Protein: 19.5 g	Carbs: 28.7 g
Fibre: 9.2 g	Total sugar: 8.5 g
Total fat: 11 g	Free sugar: 0 g

If cooking in the oven:

Preheat the oven to 180°C.

Combine the chipolatas, sweet potato, stock, mushroom, tomatoes, Worcestershire sauce, paprika and garlic in a casserole dish. Cover and bake for 40 minutes, stirring halfway. Remove the lid and cook for a further 20 minutes. Season with salt and pepper and stir through the spinach.

If cooking in a slow cooker:

Combine the chipolatas, sweet potato, stock, mushroom, tomatoes, Worcestershire sauce, paprika, garlic, salt and pepper and spinach in the slow cooker dish. Stir in 1 cup of water, then cover with the lid and cook on low for 8 hours.

To serve:

Toast the bread and place one slice on each plate. Spoon over the baked chipolatas and vegetables and serve.

Store any leftover chipolatas and vegetables in an airtight container in the fridge for 3–4 days or freeze for up to 2 months.

SUITABLE TO FREEZE

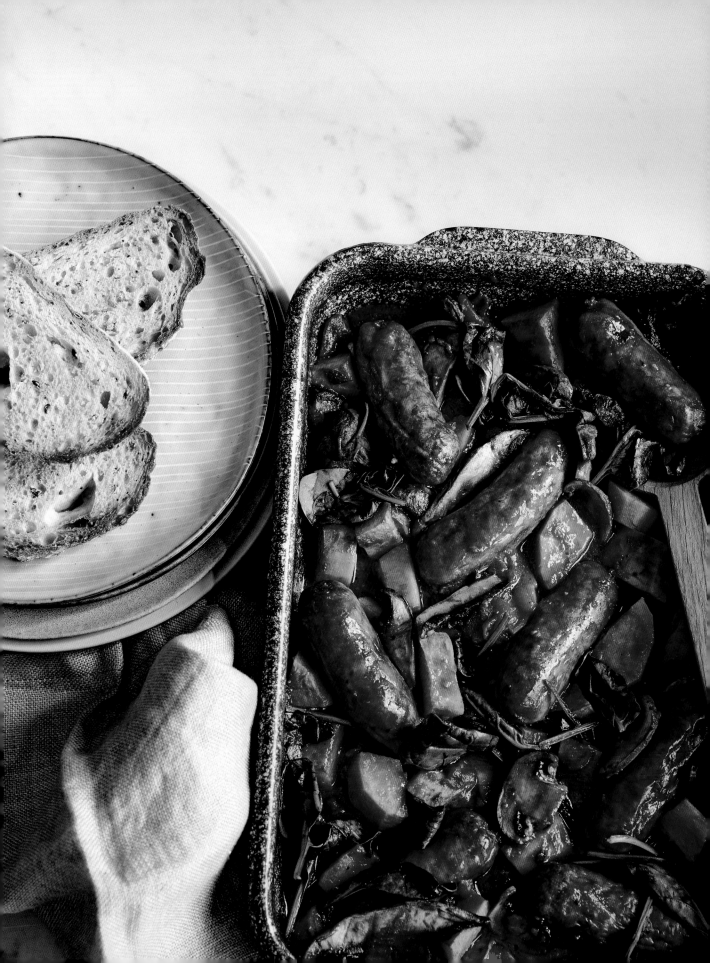

ZUCCHINI AND RICOTTA BAKE

SERVES
4

PREPARATION
10 MINS

COOK
50 MINS (8 HOURS IN
A SLOW COOKER)

COST PER SERVE
$1.71

1 teaspoon extra-virgin
   olive oil
½ brown onion, diced
1 garlic clove, crushed
2 small zucchini, diced
90 g baby spinach leaves
10 g butter
6 slices wholegrain or gluten-
   free bread of choice
½ cup reduced-fat ricotta
4 free-range eggs
1 cup reduced-fat milk
   of choice
salt and freshly ground
   black pepper
½ cup grated reduced-fat
   cheddar
½ teaspoon ground nutmeg

NUTRI DETAILS PER SERVE

1410 kJ/336 cals	Sat fat: 7 g
Protein: 22.9 g	Carbs: 23.7 g
Fibre: 4.7 g	Total sugar: 6.5 g
Total fat: 15.8 g	Free sugar: 0 g

Heat the olive oil in a frying pan over medium–high heat. Add the onion, garlic and zucchini and cook for 3–4 minutes until the onion is translucent and the zucchini is starting to turn golden. Add the spinach and stir until wilted.

Butter the bread and cut into 2 cm cubes.

If cooking in the oven:
Preheat the oven to 180°C.

Arrange the bread cubes over the base of a casserole dish, buttered-side down, and top with the zucchini and spinach mixture. Dollop the ricotta over the veggies.

Lightly beat the eggs and milk and season with salt and pepper, then pour over the ricotta and vegetables. Top with the grated cheddar and sprinkle with nutmeg.

Bake for 45 minutes until the top is golden and the egg is cooked through.

If cooking in a slow cooker:
Arrange the bread cubes over the base of the slow cooker dish, buttered-side down, and top with the zucchini and spinach mixture. Dollop the ricotta over the veggies.

Lightly beat the eggs and milk and season with salt and pepper, then pour over the ricotta and vegetables. Top with the grated cheddar and sprinkle with nutmeg.

Cook on low for 6–8 hours (or overnight).

To serve:
Divide the bake evenly among four plates and serve.

Store any leftovers in an airtight container in the fridge for 4–5 days or freeze for up to 2 months.

SUITABLE TO FREEZE

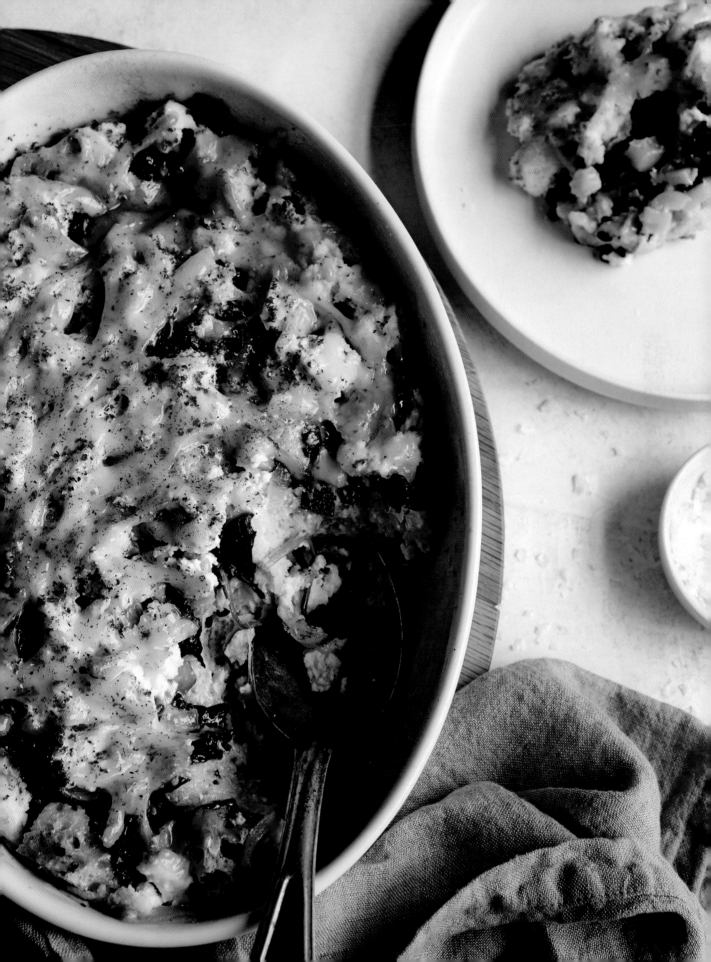

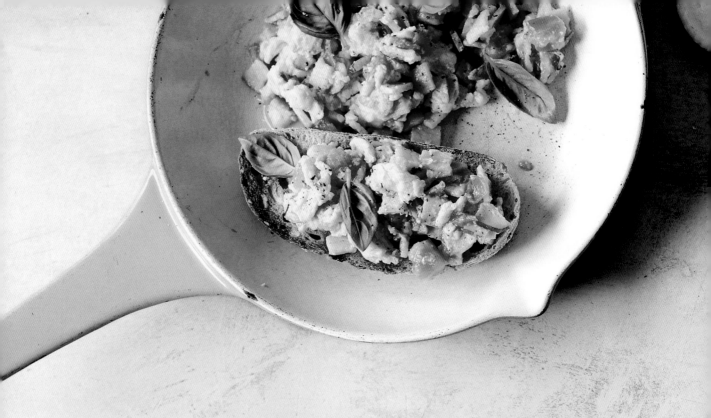

GOURMET SCRAMBLED EGGS

SERVES
1

PREPARATION
10 MINS

COOK
10 MINS

COST PER SERVE
$1.09

1 free-range egg
2 teaspoons reduced-fat milk
  of choice
cooking oil spray
2 lean bacon rashers,
  trimmed and finely diced
½ tomato, finely diced
1 slice wholegrain or gluten-
  free bread of choice
salt and freshly ground
  black pepper

NUTRI DETAILS PER SERVE

1104 kJ/263 cals	Sat fat: 3.6 g
Protein: 22.1 g	Carbs: 17 g
Fibre: 3.1 g	Total sugar: 2.7 g
Total fat: 11.1 g	Free sugar: 0 g

Lightly beat the egg and milk in a small bowl.

Spray a small frying pan with cooking oil and place over high heat. Fry the bacon for 2 minutes until golden. Add the tomato and cook for a further 2 minutes.

Reduce the heat to medium. Add the egg mixture and cook, stirring constantly, to incorporate the bacon and tomato. Remove from the heat while the egg is still softly set.

Toast the bread and immediately top with the scrambled egg. Season with salt and pepper and serve.

Tip

Serve topped with basil leaves or other fresh herbs of your choice, if you like.

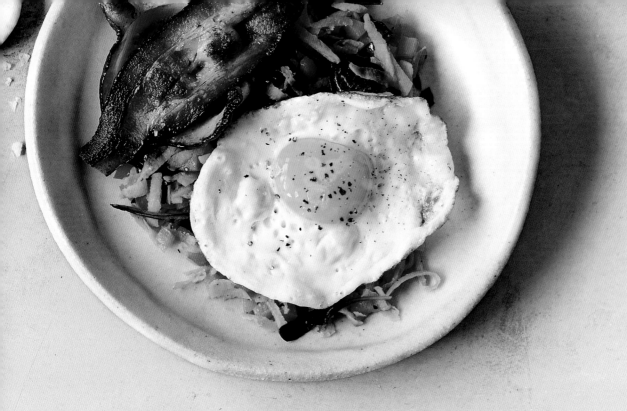

BACON AND EGG WITH VEGGIE HASH

SERVES
1

PREPARATION
5 MINS

COOK
10 MINS

COST PER SERVE
$0.99

1 teaspoon extra-virgin
   olive oil
1 lean bacon rasher, trimmed
¼ small sweet potato, grated
¼ red capsicum, finely diced
handful of baby spinach
   leaves
salt and freshly ground
   black pepper
1 free-range egg

NUTRI DETAILS PER SERVE

718 kJ/170 cals   Sat fat: 2.5 g
Protein: 11.8 g   Carbs: 6.8 g
Fibre: 1.3 g   Total sugar: 3.2 g
Total fat: 10.6 g   Free sugar: 0 g

Heat the olive oil in a frying pan over medium–high heat. Add the bacon and cook for 3–4 minutes until crunchy and golden.

Push the bacon to the side of the pan (or remove and drain on a piece of paper towel). Add the sweet potato, capsicum and spinach and cook for 3–4 minutes until the spinach has wilted and the veggies are tender. Season with salt and pepper.

Push the veggies to the side of the pan and crack in the egg. Fry for 2–3 minutes until cooked to your liking.

Serve the bacon and egg on top of the veggies.

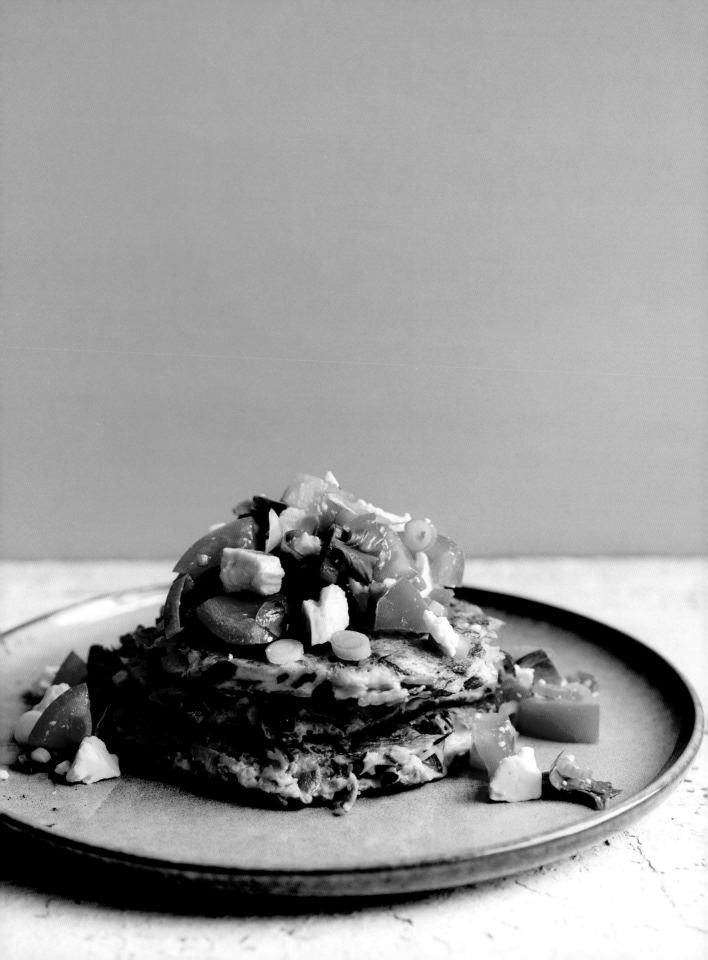

VEGGIE-LOADED FRITTERS

SERVES
1

PREPARATION
15 MINS

COOK
10 MINS

COST PER SERVE
$1.75

½ small zucchini, grated
½ carrot, grated
1 free-range egg
1 tablespoon grated
   parmesan
1 teaspoon chopped flat-leaf
   parsley leaves
salt and freshly ground
   black pepper
1 tablespoon extra-virgin
   olive oil
½ tomato, diced
1 tablespoon chopped
   basil leaves
½ garlic clove, crushed
½ spring onion, finely sliced
1 tablespoon crumbled
   reduced-fat feta

Combine the zucchini and carrot in a colander and use your hands to squeeze out any excess moisture. Place in a bowl and add the egg, parmesan and parsley. Season with salt and pepper and mix together well.

Divide the mixture into three balls and flatten.

Heat the olive oil in a frying pan over medium–high heat, add the hash browns and cook for 3–4 minutes on each side until crispy and golden. (If you are cooking more than one serve, cook them in batches.)

Meanwhile, combine the tomato, basil, garlic, spring onion and feta to make a salsa.

Serve the hash browns topped with the salsa.

NUTRI DETAILS PER SERVE

1424 kJ/339 cals	Sat fat: 7.5 g
Protein: 16 g	Carbs: 4 g
Fibre: 2.7 g	Total sugar: 3.8 g
Total fat: 28.7 g	Free sugar: 0 g

GREEK PIZZA MUFFIN

SERVES
1

PREPARATION
5 MINS

COOK
5 MINS

COST PER SERVE
$0.75

1 tablespoon tomato passata
1 wholemeal English muffin,
  split in half
⅛ red onion, diced
2 tablespoons pitted
  kalamata olives, chopped
¼ red capsicum, diced
1½ tablespoons crumbled
  reduced-fat feta
¼ teaspoon dried chilli flakes
¼ teaspoon dried oregano

Preheat an overhead grill to high.

Spread the tomato passata over both halves of the muffin and top with the onion, olives and capsicum. Sprinkle with the feta, chilli flakes and dried oregano.

Place under the grill and cook for 5 minutes until the cheese is golden and the muffin is crispy. Serve immediately.

NUTRI DETAILS PER SERVE

980 kJ/233 cals	Sat fat: 3 g
Protein: 15 g	Carbs: 28.6 g
Fibre: 3.2 g	Total sugar: 6 g
Total fat: 5.6 g	Free sugar: 0 g

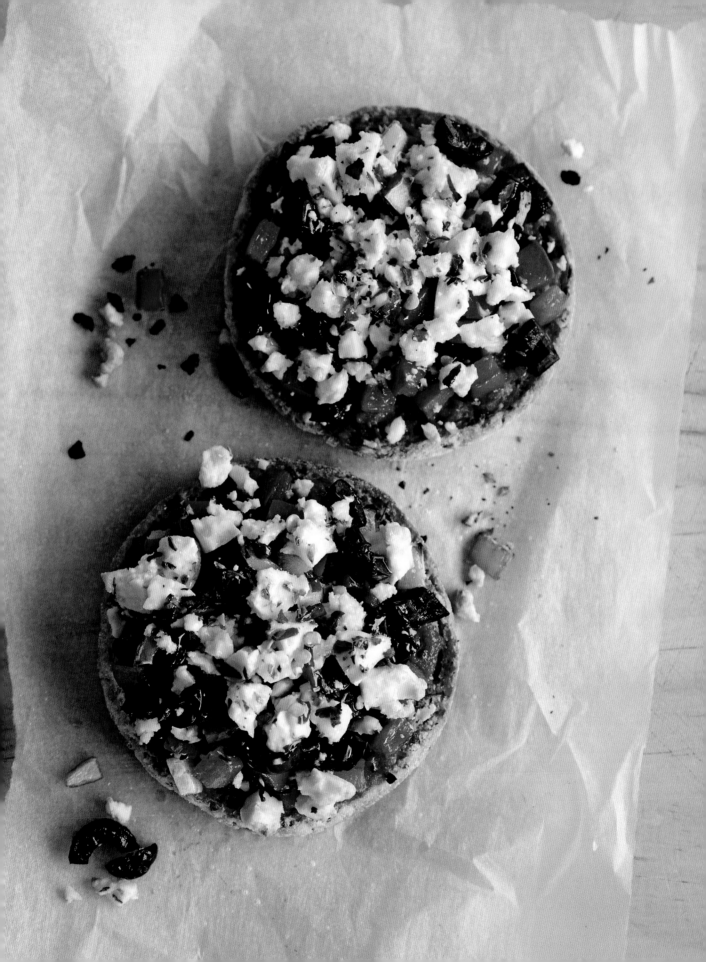

BACON AND ZUCCHINI MUFFINS

SERVES
10

PREPARATION
10 MINS

COOK
30 MINS

COST PER SERVE
$0.46

4 lean bacon rashers,
  trimmed and diced
1 small zucchini, diced
1 ¾ cups wholemeal self-
  raising flour
1 teaspoon baking powder
½ cup grated parmesan
2 free-range eggs
½ cup reduced-fat milk
  of choice
½ cup extra-virgin olive oil

NUTRI DETAILS PER SERVE

1041 kJ/248 cals	Sat fat: 3.5 g
Protein: 9.7 g	Carbs: 16.7 g
Fibre: 3 g	Total sugar: 0.9 g
Total fat: 15.3 g	Free sugar: 0 g

Preheat the oven to 200°C. Line or lightly grease 10 holes of a standard muffin tin.

Heat a non-stick frying pan over medium–high heat and add the bacon. Cook for 5 minutes until crispy and golden, then remove one-third of the bacon and set aside.

Add the zucchini to the bacon in the pan and cook for 1–2 minutes until softened. Remove from the heat.

Combine the flour, baking powder and half the parmesan in a large bowl and make a well in the centre. Crack in the eggs and pour in the milk and olive oil, then slowly bring the ingredients together until well combined.

Fold the zucchini and bacon mixture through the batter, then divide the batter evenly among the prepared muffin holes. Sprinkle the reserved bacon pieces over the top, followed by the remaining parmesan.

Bake for 15–20 minutes until a skewer inserted into the centre of a muffin comes out clean. Cool in the tin for 5 minutes before turning out onto a wire rack. Serve warm. One muffin is one serve.

Store leftover cooled muffins in an airtight container in the fridge for up to 4 days or freeze for up to 3 months.

SUITABLE TO FREEZE

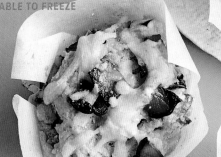

MUSHROOM AND SUN-DRIED TOMATO MINI FRITTATAS

SERVES
6

PREPARATION
10 MINS

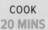

COOK
20 MINS

COST PER SERVE
$0.93

10 g butter
¼ red onion, diced
75 g mushrooms, sliced
salt and freshly ground
   black pepper
1 tablespoon chopped
   sun-dried tomatoes
1 teaspoon pine nuts, toasted
1 tablespoon chopped
   basil leaves
60 g rocket leaves, chopped
6 free-range eggs
½ cup reduced-fat cream
¼ cup grated reduced-fat
   cheddar

NUTRI DETAILS PER SERVE

676 kJ/160 cals	Sat fat: 5.7 g
Protein: 11.3 g	Carbs: 2.3 g
Fibre: 0.7 g	Total sugar: 2.2 g
Total fat: 11.9 g	Free sugar: 0 g

Preheat the oven to 180°C. Line six holes of a standard muffin tin with paper cases or baking paper.

Melt the butter in a frying pan over medium heat. Add the onion and mushroom and cook for 3–5 minutes until tender. Remove the pan from the heat. Season the onion and mushroom with salt and pepper, then stir in the sun-dried tomato, pine nuts, basil and rocket.

Lightly beat the eggs in a large bowl. Add the vegetable mixture and stir through the cream until well combined.

Divide the batter evenly among the prepared muffin holes and sprinkle the grated cheddar over the top.

Bake for 10–15 minutes until the frittatas are golden brown and a skewer inserted into the centre of a frittata comes out clean. Cool in the tin for 5 minutes before turning out onto a wire rack. Serve warm. One frittata is one serve.

Store any leftovers in an airtight container in the fridge for 3–4 days or freeze for up to 2 months.

SUITABLE TO FREEZE

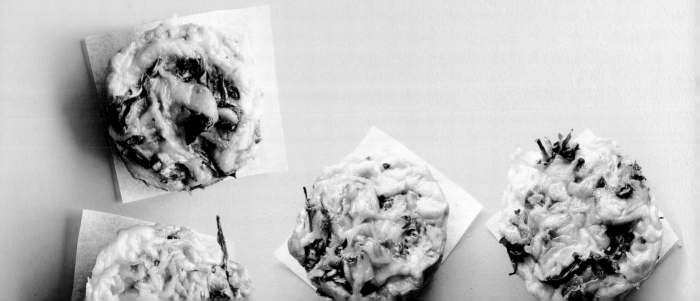

MEXICAN BREAKFAST WRAP

SERVES
1

PREPARATION
10 MINS

COOK
5 MINS

COST PER SERVE
$1.25

¼ cup canned red kidney
  beans, drained and rinsed
1 free-range egg, lightly
  beaten
1 tablespoon grated
  reduced-fat cheddar
salt and freshly ground
  black pepper
½ tomato, diced
¼ red onion, diced
1 tablespoon chopped
  coriander leaves
1 tablespoon mashed
  avocado

NUTRI DETAILS PER SERVE

928 kJ/221 cals	Sat fat: 4.3 g
Protein: 16.2 g	Carbs: 9.4 g
Fibre: 4.9 g	Total sugar: 3.3 g
Total fat: 12.2 g	Free sugar: 0 g

Heat the beans in the microwave or in a small saucepan over medium heat.

Whisk the egg, cheddar and 1 tablespoon of water in a small bowl and season with salt and pepper.

Heat a small non-stick frying pan over medium heat. Pour the egg mixture into the pan and swirl around to cover the base. Cook for 2–3 minutes until the egg is cooked through and you have a nice thin omelette.

Meanwhile, combine the tomato, onion and coriander in a bowl and season with salt and pepper.

Top the omelette with the warm beans, the tomato and onion mixture and a dollop of mashed avocado. Slide the omelette onto a plate, fold over to enclose the filling and serve.

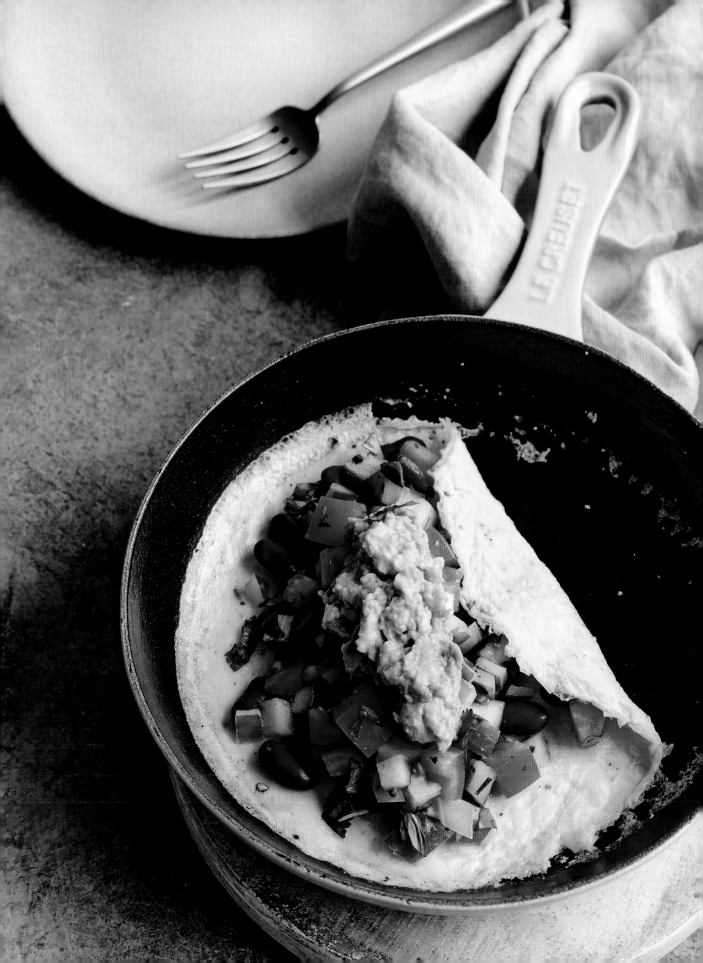

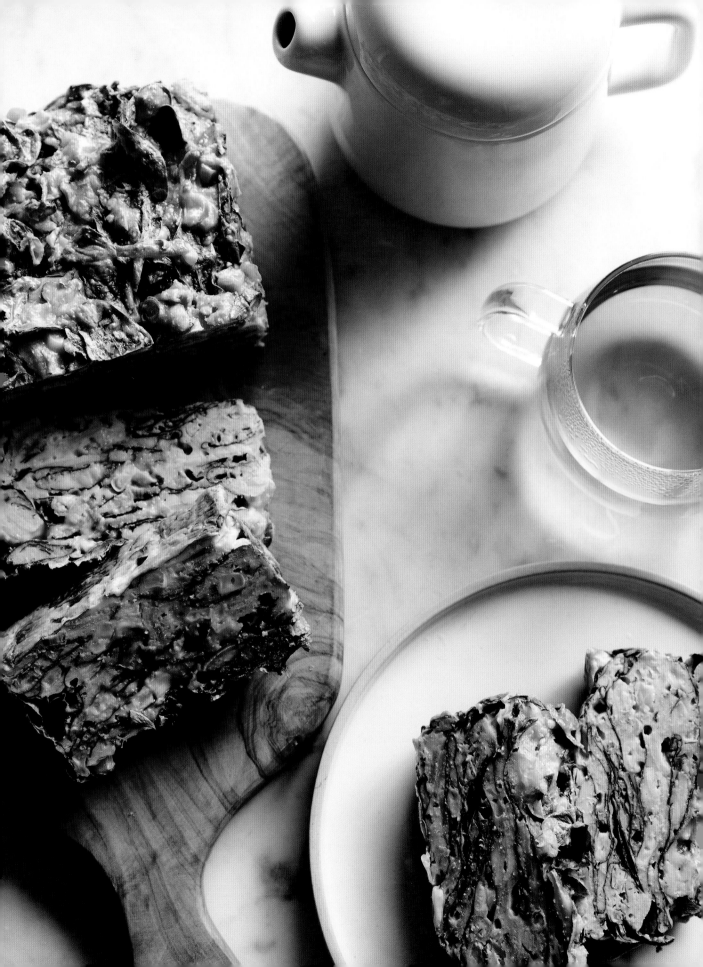

CORN AND HAM BREAKFAST SLICE

SERVES
4

PREPARATION
10 MINS

COOK
25 MINS

COST PER SERVE
$1.47

cooking oil spray
1 cup corn kernels (fresh
    or canned)
6 free-range eggs,
    lightly beaten
4 slices lean smoked ham,
    diced
1 cup wholemeal self-raising
    flour
⅓ cup grated reduced-fat
    cheddar
1 spring onion, finely sliced
120 g baby spinach leaves,
    chopped
salt and freshly ground
    black pepper

Preheat the oven to 180°C. Lightly spray a standard loaf tin with cooking oil.

Combine all the ingredients in a bowl and season with salt and pepper. Pour the batter into the prepared tin and bake for 20–25 minutes until the slice is cooked and firm.

Cut into four pieces and serve. One piece is one serve.

Store any leftovers in an airtight container in the fridge for 3–4 days or freeze in portions for up to 2 months.

SUITABLE TO FREEZE

NUTRI DETAILS PER SERVE

1364 kJ/325 cals
Protein: 22 g
Fibre: 4.8 g
Total fat: 13 g

Sat fat: 5.5 g
Carbs: 28 g
Total sugar: 2.5 g
Free sugar: 0 g

HAWAIIAN MELTS

SERVES
1

PREPARATION
5 MINS

COOK
5 MINS

COST PER SERVE
$2.23

---

2 slices wholegrain or gluten-free bread of choice
3 slices lean smoked ham
2 pineapple rings (fresh or canned)
2 teaspoons chopped sun-dried tomatoes
⅛ teaspoon smoked paprika
⅓ cup grated reduced-fat cheddar
small handful of baby spinach leaves

NUTRI DETAILS PER SERVE

1394 kJ/332 cals
Protein: 28.5 g
Fibre: 5 g
Total fat: 10.7 g

Sat fat: 5 g
Carbs: 27.6 g
Total sugar: 10.5 g
Free sugar: 0 g

Preheat an overhead grill to medium–high.

Place the bread slices under the grill for a minute or so until one side is golden. Remove from the grill. Top the untoasted side of each piece with ham, a pineapple ring, some sun-dried tomato, a sprinkle of paprika and the grated cheese.

Return to the grill and cook for 1–2 minutes until the cheese is melted and golden. Scatter the baby spinach on top of each slice, cut them in half and serve immediately.

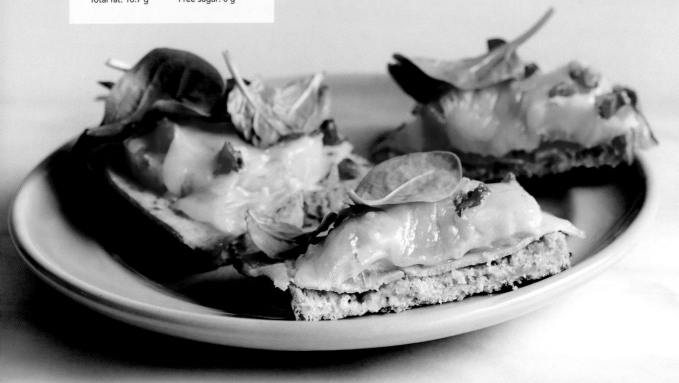

TURMERIC EGG AND BACON WRAP

SERVES
1

PREPARATION
5 MINS

COOK
10 MINS

COST PER SERVE
$1.99

2 free-range eggs
¼ teaspoon ground turmeric
1 tablespoon chopped flat-leaf parsley leaves
2 lean bacon rashers, trimmed
30 g rocket leaves
1 wholemeal mountain bread wrap

NUTRI DETAILS PER SERVE

1382 kJ/329 cals	Sat fat: 5.4 g
Protein: 30.1 g	Carbs: 14.2 g
Fibre: 2.3 g	Total sugar: 2.7 g
Total fat: 16.7 g	Free sugar: 0 g

Lightly beat the eggs, turmeric and parsley in a bowl, then pour into a non-stick frying pan and heat over medium–high heat. Cook, moving the egg around constantly to ensure it doesn't stick, for 3–4 minutes until cooked to your liking.

Meanwhile, place the bacon in a separate non-stick frying pan over high heat and cook for about 3 minutes on each side. (Alternatively, place the bacon on a lined baking tray and cook under an overhead grill preheated to high.)

Place the rocket on the mountain bread wrap, layer on the egg and bacon, then wrap and enjoy.

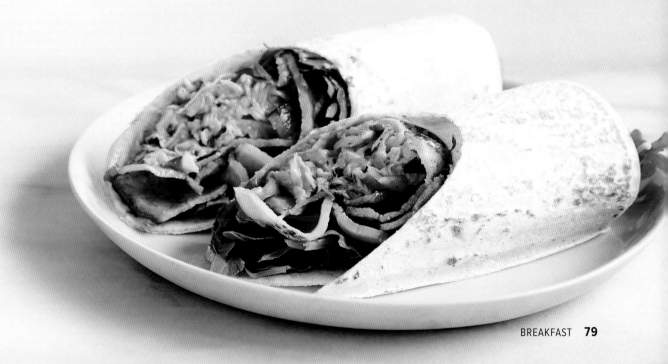

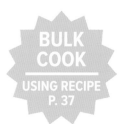

BULK COOK

USING RECIPE
P. 37

ROASTED RAINBOW VEGGIE BREAKFAST SALAD

SERVES
4

PREPARATION
5 MINS

COOK
10 MINS, PLUS
BASE RECIPE

COST PER SERVE
$2.50

- **1 x quantity Roasted Rainbow Veggies (see p. 37)**
- **2 teaspoons white vinegar**
- **4 free-range eggs**
- **120 g baby spinach leaves**
- **1 teaspoon organic hemp seeds**

NUTRI DETAILS PER SERVE

1400 kJ/333 cals	Sat fat: 3 g
Protein: 15.6 g	Carbs: 28.8 g
Fibre: 8.8 g	Total sugar: 16.9 g
Total fat: 15.6 g	Free sugar: 0 g

Reheat the roasted rainbow veggies in the microwave or on the stovetop until warmed through.

Meanwhile, fill a medium saucepan with water until three-quarters full and bring to the boil over medium–high heat. Add the vinegar and reduce the heat to medium–low. Crack each egg into a small bowl. Use a spoon to stir the water to make a whirlpool, then carefully add one egg at a time to the centre of the whirlpool. Cook for 3 minutes for soft yolks or 4 minutes or so for firm yolks. Remove the eggs with a slotted spoon and drain on paper towel.

Toss the baby spinach through the roasted rainbow veggies and divide among four bowls. Top each bowl with a poached egg and a sprinkle of hemp seeds and serve.

Store any leftover roasted rainbow veggies in an airtight container in the fridge for 3–4 days or freeze for up to 3 months.

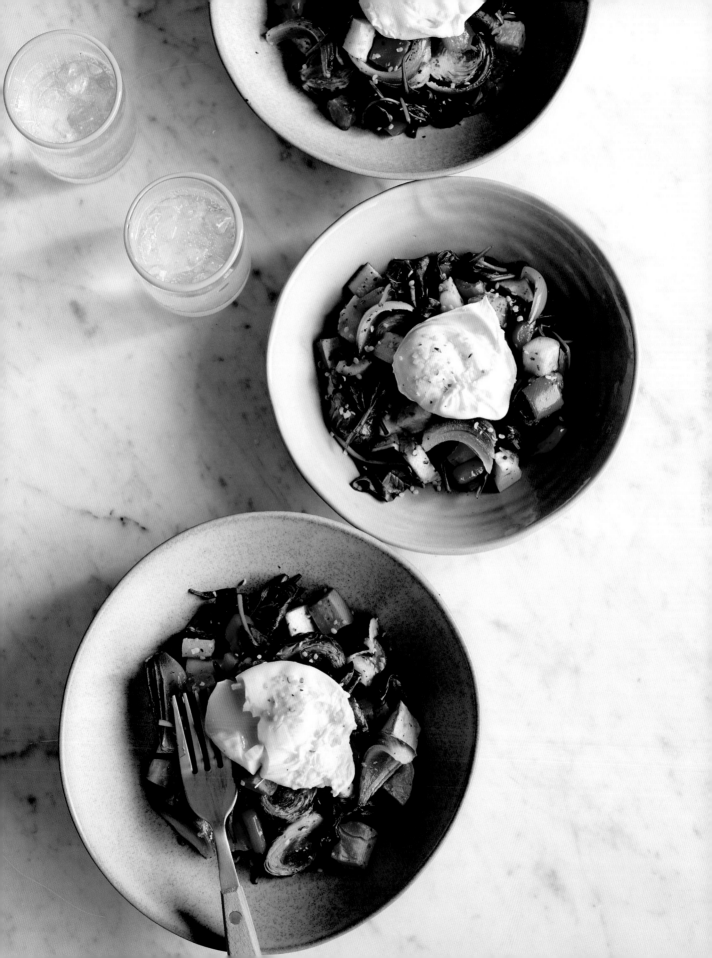

SMOOTHIES

Meals on the go!

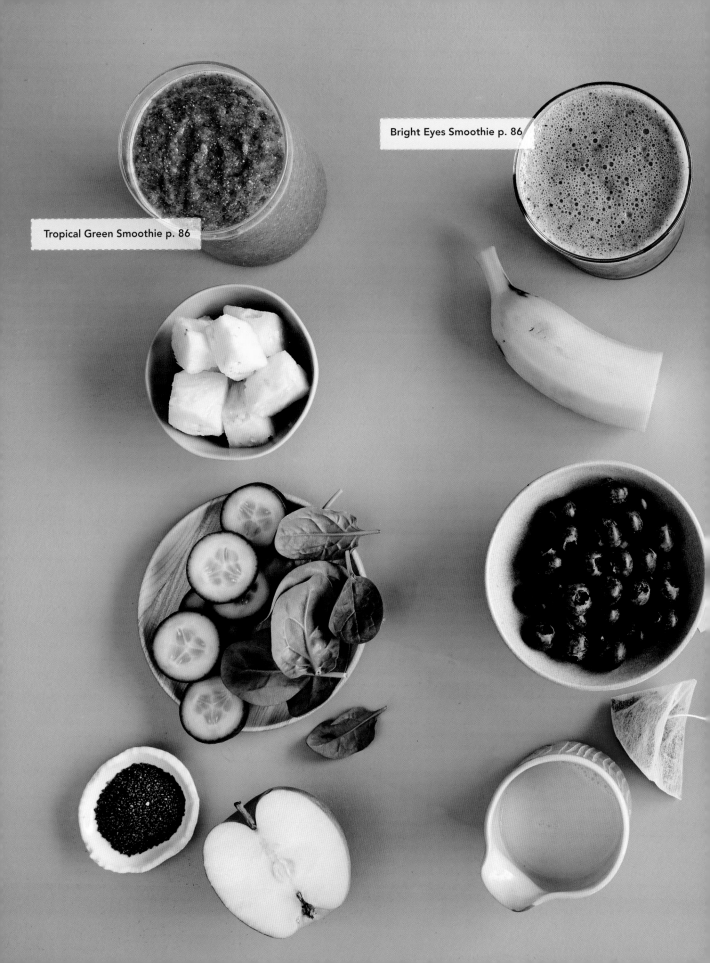

Tropical Green Smoothie p. 86

Bright Eyes Smoothie p. 86

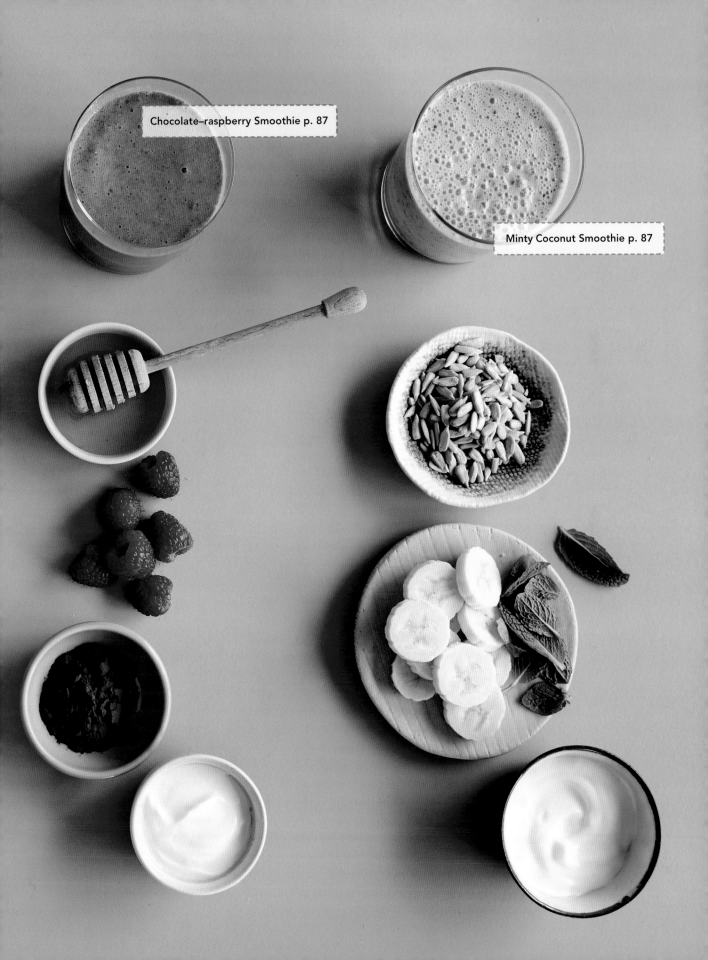

Chocolate–raspberry Smoothie p. 87

Minty Coconut Smoothie p. 87

TROPICAL GREEN SMOOTHIE

SERVES
1

PREPARATION
5 MINS

COST PER SERVE
$2.35

¼ Lebanese cucumber, chopped
1 small apple, chopped
handful of baby spinach leaves
½ cup chopped pineapple (fresh or canned)
1 tablespoon chia seeds
1 cup coconut water

Place all the ingredients in a blender and blitz until smooth. Pour into a glass and serve.

NUTRI DETAILS PER SERVE

810 kJ/193 cals
Protein: 6 g
Fibre: 9.7 g
Total fat: 5.4 g

Sat fat: 1 g
Carbs: 29.2 g
Total sugar: 22.3 g
Free sugar: 0 g

BRIGHT EYES SMOOTHIE

SERVES
1

PREPARATION
10 MINS

COST PER SERVE
$2.43

1 green teabag
½ cup boiling water
½ cup blueberries (fresh or frozen)
½ small banana
1 cup unsweetened almond milk
ice cubes

Place the teabag in a mug and pour over the boiling water. Allow to steep for 3 minutes, then remove the teabag. Set aside to cool.

Place the cooled tea and all the remaining ingredients in a blender and blitz until smooth. Pour into a glass and serve.

NUTRI DETAILS PER SERVE

736 kJ/175 cals
Protein: 74.1 g
Fibre: 3.1 g
Total fat: 4.8 g

Sat fat: 0.5 g
Carbs: 28.7 g
Total sugar: 23 g
Free sugar: 0 g

CHOCOLATE–RASPBERRY SMOOTHIE

SERVES
1

PREPARATION
5 MINS

COST PER SERVE
$1.44

1 teaspoon cacao powder
½ cup raspberries (fresh or frozen)
1 teaspoon chia seeds
1 cup reduced-fat milk of choice
1 tablespoon reduced-fat plain
   Greek yoghurt
1 teaspoon honey

Place all the ingredients in a blender and blitz until smooth. Pour into a glass and serve.

NUTRI DETAILS PER SERVE

1023 kJ/243 cals	Sat fat: 3 g
Protein: 13.5 g	Carbs: 29.8 g
Fibre: 7.9 g	Total sugar: 27 g
Total fat: 6.3 g	Free sugar: 5.8 g

MINTY COCONUT SMOOTHIE

SERVES
1

PREPARATION
5 MINS

COST PER SERVE
$1.55

½ small banana
2 tablespoons mint leaves
¼ cup reduced-fat plain Greek yoghurt
1 tablespoon sunflower seeds
1 cup coconut water

Place all the ingredients in a blender and blitz until smooth. Pour into a glass and serve.

NUTRI DETAILS PER SERVE

873 kJ/208 cals	Sat fat: 1.9 g
Protein: 9.8 g	Carbs: 17.9 g
Fibre: 3.4 g	Total sugar: 16.2 g
Total fat: 9.9 g	Free sugar: 0 g

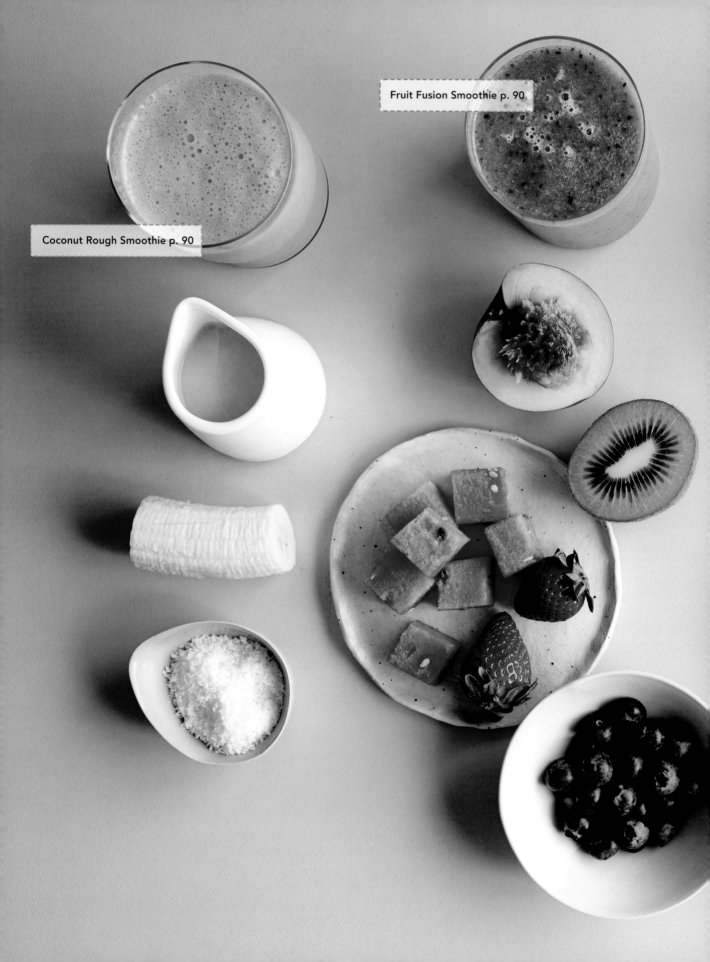

Coconut Rough Smoothie p. 90

Fruit Fusion Smoothie p. 90

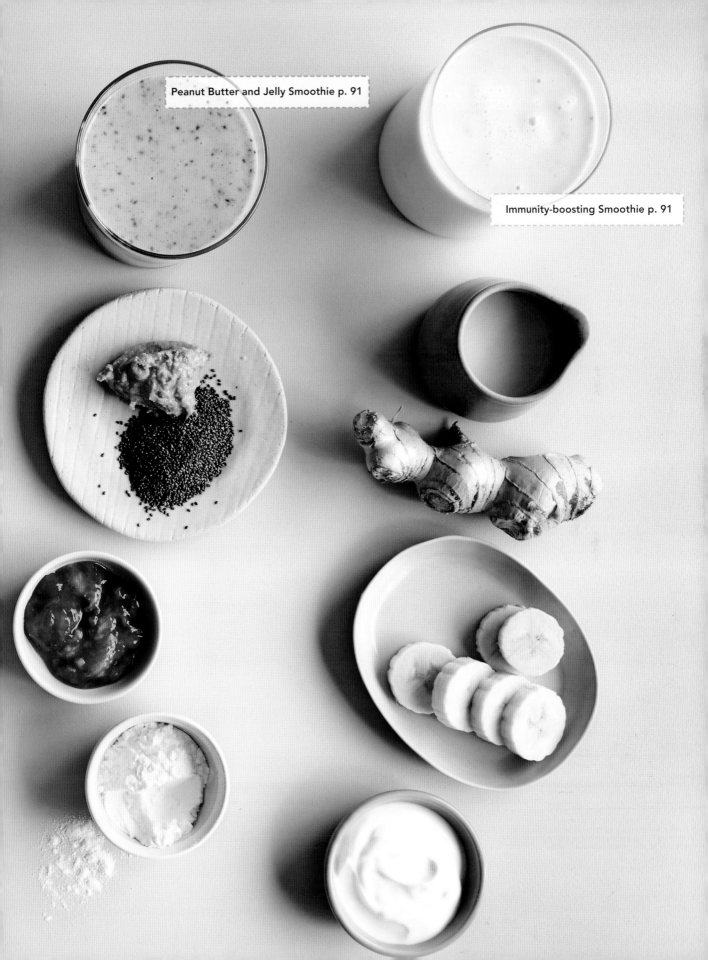

Peanut Butter and Jelly Smoothie p. 91

Immunity-boosting Smoothie p. 91

COCONUT ROUGH SMOOTHIE

SERVES	PREPARATION	COST PER SERVE
1	5 MINS	$1.16

1 tablespoon desiccated coconut
1 cup low-fat chocolate-flavoured soy milk
½ frozen banana
ice cubes

Place all the ingredients in a blender and blitz until smooth. Pour into a glass and serve.

NUTRI DETAILS PER SERVE

853 kJ/ 203 cals	Sat fat: 4.8 g
Protein: 10.4 g	Carbs: 24.5 g
Fibre: 3.5 g	Total sugar: 13.5 g
Total fat: 6.5 g	Free sugar: 5 g

FRUIT FUSION SMOOTHIE

SERVES	PREPARATION	COST PER SERVE
1	5 MINS	$2.50

½ kiwi fruit, peeled and chopped
1 slice watermelon, chopped
1 small nectarine, stone removed
¼ cup blueberries (fresh or frozen)
65 g strawberries, hulled and chopped
1 cup coconut water

Place all the ingredients in a blender and blitz until smooth. Pour into a glass and serve.

NUTRI DETAILS PER SERVE

656 kJ/156 cals	Sat fat: 0.5 g
Protein: 5.3 g	Carbs: 27.6 g
Fibre: 7.1 g	Total sugar: 27.4 g
Total fat: 0.9 g	Free sugar: 0 g

PEANUT BUTTER AND JELLY SMOOTHIE

SERVES 1

PREPARATION 5 MINS

COST PER SERVE $2.49

2 tablespoons strawberry smoothie powder of choice (see Tip)
1 tablespoon peanut butter
1 teaspoon sugar-free strawberry jam
¼ teaspoon ground cinnamon
2 teaspoons chia seeds
¾ cup reduced-fat milk of choice

Place all the ingredients and ½ cup of water in a blender and blitz until smooth. Pour into a glass and serve.

Check out The Healthy Mummy range of smoothie powders at healthymummy.com

NUTRI DETAILS PER SERVE

946 kJ/225 cals	Sat fat: 1.7 g
Protein: 19.5 g	Carbs: 7.1 g
Fibre: 6.2 g	Total sugar: 1.2 g
Total fat: 12.4 g	Free sugar: 0 g

IMMUNITY-BOOSTING SMOOTHIE

SERVES 1

PREPARATION 5 MINS

COST PER SERVE $2.44

2 tablespoons vanilla smoothie powder of choice (see Tip)
½ small banana
1 tablespoon reduced-fat plain Greek yoghurt
½ cup unsweetened almond milk
¼ teaspoon grated ginger

Place all the ingredients and ½ cup of water in a blender and blitz until smooth. Pour into a glass and serve.

NUTRI DETAILS PER SERVE

762 kJ/ 181 cals	Sat fat: 0.6 g
Protein: 51.8 g	Carbs: 17 g
Fibre: 2.7 g	Total sugar: 11.7 g
Total fat: 4.3 g	Free sugar: 0 g

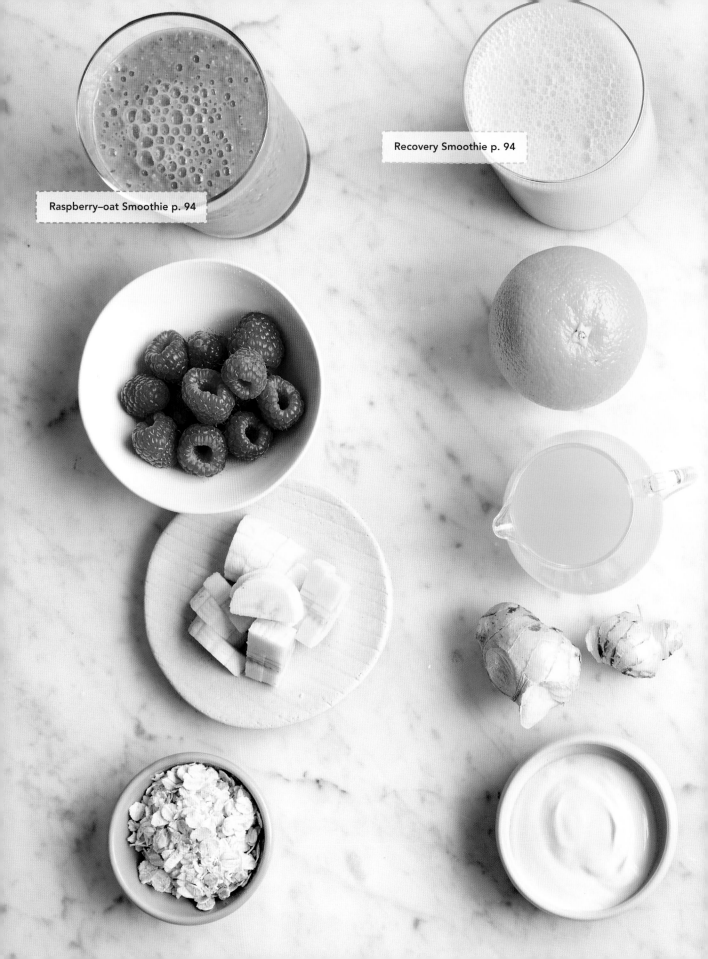

Raspberry–oat Smoothie p. 94

Recovery Smoothie p. 94

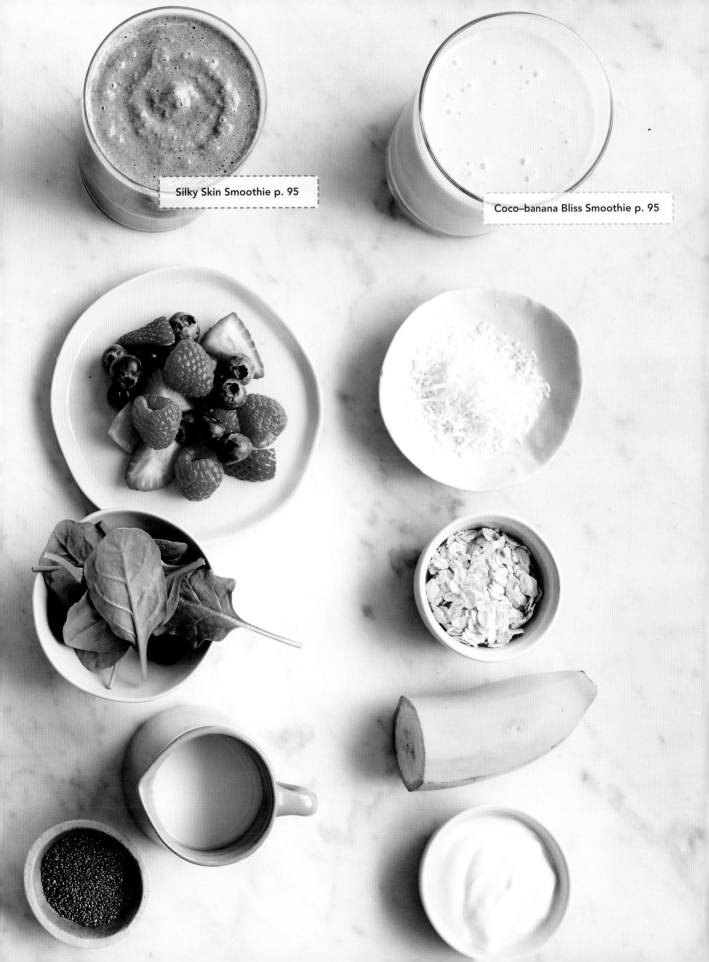

Silky Skin Smoothie p. 95

Coco–banana Bliss Smoothie p. 95

RASPBERRY–OAT SMOOTHIE

SERVES
1

PREPARATION
5 MINS

COST PER SERVE
$2.12

½ small banana
½ cup raspberries (fresh or frozen)
2 tablespoons rolled oats
1 cup coconut water

Place all the ingredients in a blender and blitz until smooth. Pour into a glass and serve.

NUTRI DETAILS PER SERVE

760 kJ/181 cals
Protein: 5.7 g
Fibre: 8.5 g
Total fat: 2.4 g

Sat fat: 0.7 g
Carbs: 29.1 g
Total sugar: 17.3 g
Free sugar: 0 g

RECOVERY SMOOTHIE

SERVES
1

PREPARATION
5 MINS

COST PER SERVE
$1.01

1 orange, peeled
¼ cup reduced-fat plain Greek yoghurt
1 cup unsweetened pineapple juice
1 teaspoon grated ginger
ice cubes

Place all the ingredients and ½ cup of water in a blender and blitz until smooth. Pour into a glass and serve.

NUTRI DETAILS PER SERVE

907 kJ/ 216 cals
Protein: 5.6 g
Fibre: 2.6 g
Total fat: 1.5 g

Sat fat: 0.7 g
Carbs: 42.7 g
Total sugar: 42.7 g
Free sugar: 27 g

SILKY SKIN SMOOTHIE

SERVES
1

PREPARATION
5 MINS

COST PER SERVE
$1.64

30 g baby spinach leaves
½ cup mixed berries (fresh or frozen)
1 tablespoon chia seeds
1 cup reduced-fat milk of choice
ice cubes

Place all the ingredients in a blender and blitz until smooth. Pour into a glass and serve.

NUTRI DETAILS PER SERVE

937 kJ/223 cals	Sat fat: 2.8 g
Protein: 14.5 g	Carbs: 22.5 g
Fibre: 7.6 g	Total sugar: 16.1 g
Total fat: 8.4 g	Free sugar: 0 g

COCO–BANANA BLISS SMOOTHIE

SERVES
1

PREPARATION
5 MINS

COST PER SERVE
$2.45

2 tablespoons vanilla smoothie powder
  of choice (see Tip)
1 cup reduced-fat milk of choice
½ small banana
1 tablespoon shredded coconut
1 tablespoon rolled oats
1 tablespoon reduced-fat plain
  Greek yoghurt

Place all the ingredients in a blender and blitz until smooth. Pour into a glass and serve.

Check out The Healthy Mummy range of smoothie powders at healthymummy.com

NUTRI DETAILS PER SERVE

1520 kJ/362 cals	Sat fat: 8.5 g
Protein: 27 g	Carbs: 32.1 g
Fibre: 4.6 g	Total sugar: 23.8 g
Total fat: 12.9 g	Free sugar: 0 g

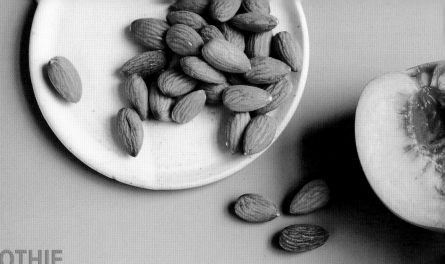

ENERGISING SMOOTHIE

SERVES
1

PREPARATION
5 MINS

COST PER SERVE
$2.48

2 tablespoons chocolate smoothie powder
  of choice (see Tip)
½ cup reduced-fat milk of choice
1 teaspoon instant coffee granules
1 teaspoon ground cinnamon
1 tablespoon chopped almonds
1 tablespoon rolled oats

Place all the ingredients and ½ cup of water
in a blender and blitz until smooth. Pour into
a glass and serve.

 Tip

Check out The Healthy Mummy range of smoothie
powders at healthymummy.com

NUTRI DETAILS PER SERVE	
1026 kJ/244cals	Sat fat: 1.7 g
Protein: 22 g	Carbs: 15 g
Fibre: 3.7 g	Total sugar: 7.7 g
Total fat: 9.7 g	Free sugar: 0 g

Energising Smoothie

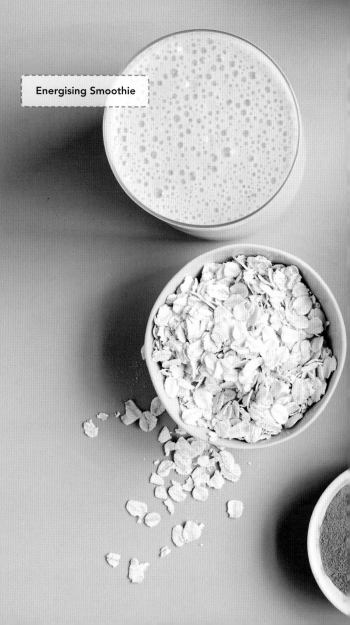

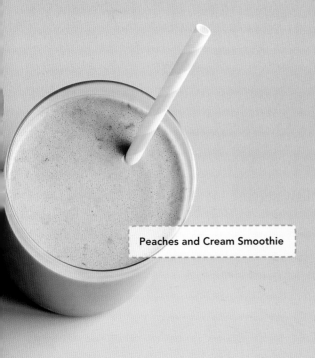

Peaches and Cream Smoothie

PEACHES AND CREAM SMOOTHIE

SERVES	PREPARATION	COST PER SERVE
1	5 MINS	$1.27

1 peach, stone removed
2 tablespoons reduced-fat plain
  Greek yoghurt
½ teaspoon ground cinnamon
1 cup reduced-fat milk of choice
ice cubes

Place all the ingredients in a blender and blitz until smooth. Pour into a glass and serve.

NUTRI DETAILS PER SERVE

855 kJ/203 cals	Sat fat: 2.8 g
Protein: 13.4 g	Carbs: 26 g
Fibre: 2 g	Total sugar: 25.8 g
Total fat: 4.4 g	Free sugar: 0 g

Mango–passionfruit Smoothie

MANGO–PASSIONFRUIT SMOOTHIE

SERVES	PREPARATION	COST PER SERVE
1	5 MINS	$1.96

1 cheek fresh or frozen mango
2 tablespoons passionfruit pulp
1 cup coconut water

Place all the ingredients in a blender and blitz until smooth. Pour into a glass and serve.

NUTRI DETAILS PER SERVE

469 kJ/112 cals	Sat fat: 0.5 g
Protein: 4 g	Carbs: 17.9 g
Fibre: 7 g	Total sugar: 17.4 g
Total fat: 0.8 g	Free sugar: 0 g

SALADS & LIGHT MEALS

Lunch options sorted!

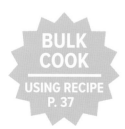

BULK COOK
USING RECIPE
P. 37

ROASTED RAINBOW VEGGIE, KALE AND QUINOA SALAD

SERVES
4

PREPARATION
5 MINS

COOK
15 MINS, PLUS
BASE RECIPE

COST PER SERVE
$2.14

½ cup quinoa, rinsed
1 x quantity Roasted Rainbow
Veggies (see p. 37)
30 g kale leaves, shredded
1 tablespoon pumpkin seeds,
toasted

NUTRI DETAILS PER SERVE

1520 kJ/362 cals	Sat fat: 1.8 g
Protein: 13 g	Carbs: 44.7 g
Fibre: 10.8 g	Total sugar: 17 g
Total fat: 12.8 g	Free sugar: 0

Place the quinoa and 1 cup of water in a small saucepan and bring to the boil. Reduce the heat and simmer, covered, for 15 minutes until tender and most of the liquid has been absorbed. Fluff up with a fork, then set aside to cool.

Meanwhile, reheat the roasted rainbow veggies in the microwave or on the stovetop until warmed through.

Combine the quinoa, roasted rainbow veggies and kale in a bowl.

Divide the salad evenly among four bowls, sprinkle with the pumpkin seeds and serve.

Store any leftover roasted rainbow veggies in an airtight container in the fridge for 3–4 days or freeze for up to 3 months.

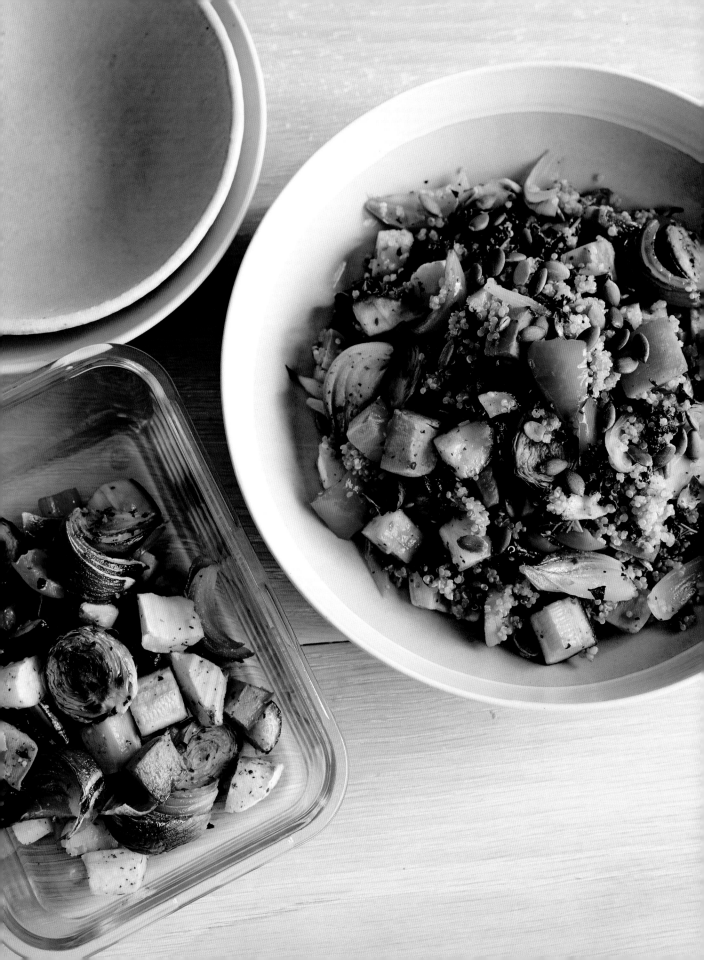

TUNA, ROASTED PUMPKIN AND BROWN RICE SALAD

SERVES
1

PREPARATION
10 MINS, PLUS
COOLING TIME

COOK
25 MINS

COST PER SERVE
$1.70

1½ tablespoons brown rice
120 g pumpkin, peeled and
  seeds removed, cubed
cooking oil spray
2 teaspoons reduced-fat plain
  Greek yoghurt
1 teaspoon reduced-fat
  mayonnaise
¼ garlic clove, crushed
1 teaspoon lemon juice
1 x 95 g can tuna in spring
  water, drained
1 tablespoon chopped
  walnuts
½ tomato, chopped
½ spring onion, finely sliced
small handful of rocket leaves

Bring 2 cups of water to the boil in a medium saucepan, add the rice and simmer for 25 minutes until tender. Drain and set aside to cool slightly. You could use pre-cooked rice for this recipe if you have some on hand. Just warm it through first.

Meanwhile, preheat the oven to 180°C and line a baking tray with baking paper.

Spread the pumpkin over the prepared tray in a single layer and spray with cooking oil. Roast for 20–25 minutes until tender and golden. Set aside to cool slightly.

Place the yoghurt, mayonnaise, garlic and lemon juice in a bowl and mix together well.

Combine the pumpkin, rice, tuna, walnuts, tomato and spring onion in a bowl. Drizzle over the yoghurt dressing, toss well to combine, top with the rocket leaves and serve.

NUTRI DETAILS PER SERVE

1475 kJ/351 cals	Sat fat: 2 g
Protein: 29.6 g	Carbs: 31.5 g
Fibre: 4.7 g	Total sugar: 9.3 g
Total fat: 10.7 g	Free sugar: 0 g

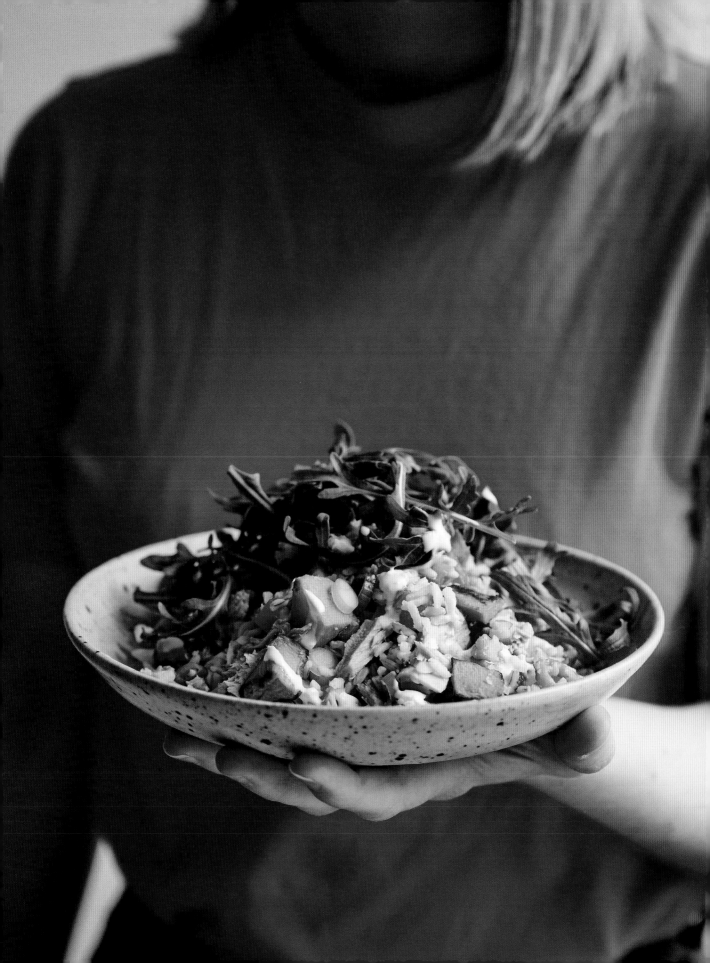

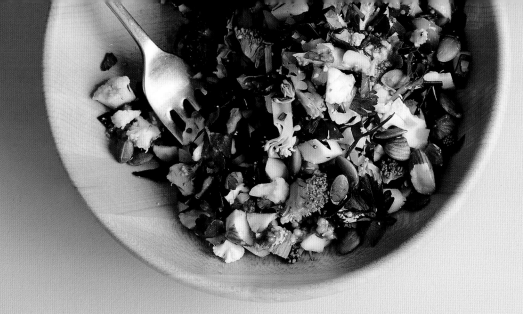

REFRESHING DETOX SALAD

SERVES
1

PREPARATION
10 MINS

COST PER SERVE
$1.23

50 g cauliflower
50 g broccoli
25 g red cabbage
½ carrot
¼ cup chopped flat-leaf
   parsley leaves
1½ tablespoons chopped
   almonds
1½ tablespoons pumpkin
   seeds, toasted
1 teaspoon extra-virgin
   olive oil
1 teaspoon lemon juice
⅛ teaspoon ground ginger
1 small garlic clove, crushed
1 teaspoon wholegrain
   mustard

Place the cauliflower, broccoli, cabbage and carrot in a food processor and blitz to grate or chop to your desired style. Remove and place in a bowl with the parsley, almonds and pumpkin seeds.

Place the olive oil, lemon juice, ginger, garlic and mustard in a jar and shake to combine. Alternatively, whisk together in a small bowl.

Drizzle the dressing over the salad and serve.

NUTRI DETAILS PER SERVE

1344 kJ/320 cals	Sat fat: 2.6 g
Protein: 13.5 g	Carbs: 8.5 g
Fibre: 10.5 g	Total sugar: 5.5 g
Total fat: 23.9 g	Free sugar: 0 g

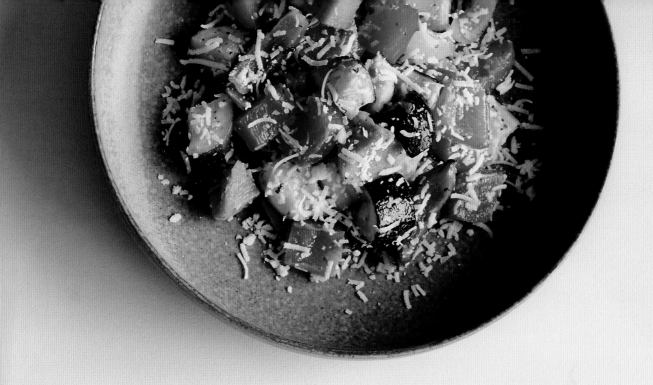

SIMPLE ROASTED VEGGIE SALAD

SERVES
1

PREPARATION
10 MINS

COOK
25 MINS

COST PER SERVE
$1.22

½ small zucchini, chopped
½ red capsicum, chopped
60 g pumpkin, peeled and
   seeds removed, cubed
⅛ red onion, diced
2 teaspoons extra-virgin
   olive oil
1 garlic clove, crushed
2 tablespoons grated
   parmesan

Preheat the oven to 180°C and line a baking tray with baking paper.

Spread the zucchini, capsicum, pumpkin and onion over the prepared tray in a single layer. Drizzle over the olive oil and toss to combine. Roast for 20–25 minutes until the vegetables are tender.

Toss the garlic through the roasted vegetables and serve sprinkled with the parmesan.

NUTRI DETAILS PER SERVE

1135 kJ/271 cals	Sat fat: 8.9 g
Protein: 15.4 g	Carbs: 2.8 g
Fibre: 1.9 g	Total sugar: 2.5 g
Total fat: 21.9 g	Free sugar: 0 g

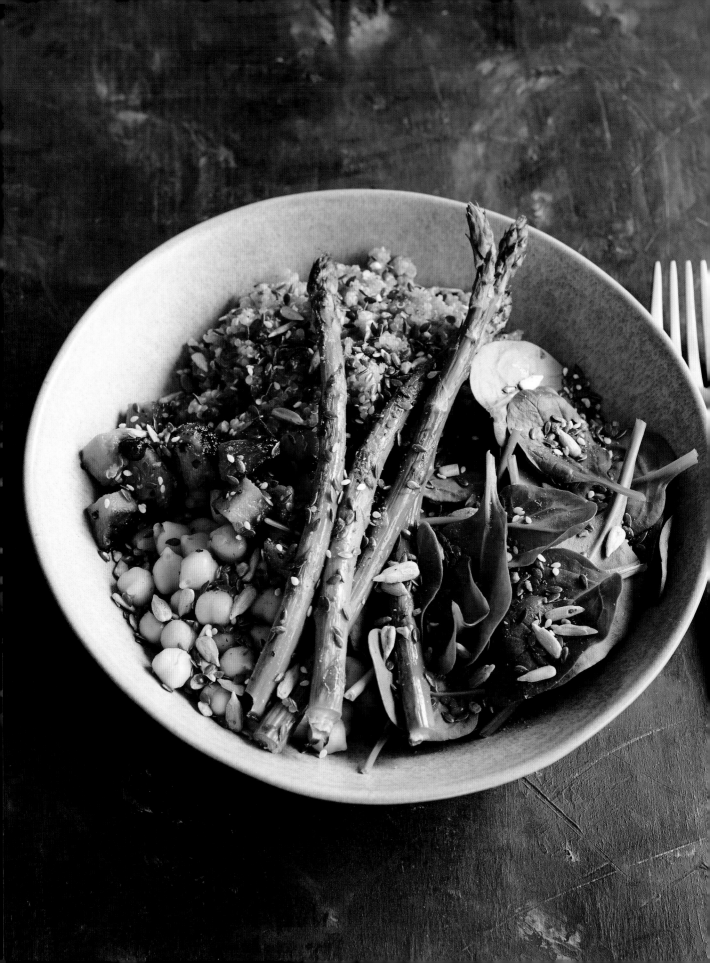

BUDDHA BOWL

SERVES
1

PREPARATION
10 MINS

COOK
25 MINS

COST PER SERVE
$2.50

---

60 g pumpkin, peeled and
  seeds removed, cubed
cooking oil spray
¼ bunch asparagus, woody
  ends trimmed
¼ cup quinoa, rinsed
handful of baby spinach
  leaves
80 g canned chickpeas,
  drained and rinsed
1 teaspoon dukkah (Middle
  Eastern seed and spice mix)
2 teaspoons sunflower seeds
1 tablespoon linseeds

NUTRI DETAILS PER SERVE

1587 kJ/378 cals	Sat fat: 1.4 g
Protein: 17 g	Carbs: 48.6 g
Fibre: 11 g	Total sugar: 3.9 g
Total fat: 12.3 g	Free sugar: 0 g

Preheat the oven to 180°C and line a baking tray with baking paper.

Spread the pumpkin over the prepared tray in a single layer and lightly spray with cooking oil. Roast for 20–25 minutes until tender and golden. About 5 minutes before the pumpkin is ready, add the asparagus to the tray for the remaining cooking time.

Meanwhile, place the quinoa and ½ cup of water in a small saucepan and bring to the boil. Reduce the heat and simmer, covered, for 15 minutes until tender and most of the liquid has been absorbed. Fluff up with a fork, then set aside to cool slightly.

Place the baby spinach, chickpeas, quinoa and pumpkin in separate sections of a bowl and arrange the asparagus on top. Sprinkle over the dukkah, sunflower seeds and linseeds and serve.

SPICED CHICKPEA BOWL

SERVES
1

PREPARATION
20 MINS

COOK
20 MINS

COST PER SERVE
$1.95

¼ red onion, cut into wedges
½ small sweet potato, peeled
  and cut into 2 cm cubes
cooking oil spray
100 g broccoli, cut into florets
30 g kale leaves, shredded
200 g canned chickpeas,
  drained and rinsed
½ teaspoon ground cumin
¼ teaspoon chilli powder
¼ teaspoon garlic powder
¼ teaspoon dried oregano
¼ teaspoon ground turmeric
1 tablespoon tahini
1 teaspoon pure maple syrup
1 tablespoon lemon juice
splash of hot water (optional)

NUTRI DETAILS PER SERVE

1715 kJ/410 cals	Sat fat: 1.5 g
Protein: 16.8 g	Carbs: 65.3 g
Fibre: 17.3 g	Total sugar: 15.8 g
Total fat: 12 g	Free sugar: 2 g

Preheat the oven to 180°C and line a baking tray with baking paper.

Spread the onion and sweet potato over the prepared tray in a single layer and lightly spray with cooking oil. Roast for 15–20 minutes until tender and golden.

Meanwhile, steam the broccoli on the stovetop or in the microwave until tender crisp. Add the kale for the last few minutes and steam until tender.

Heat a frying pan over medium–high heat, add the chickpeas, cumin, chilli powder, garlic powder, dried oregano and turmeric and toss well to combine. Dry-roast for 4–5 minutes until the chickpeas are golden and well combined with the seasonings.

Whisk the tahini, maple syrup and lemon juice in a bowl, adding a little hot water, if required, to reach a thin consistency.

Place the sweet potato and onion, broccoli, kale and spiced chickpeas in separate sections of a bowl. Drizzle over the tahini sauce and serve.

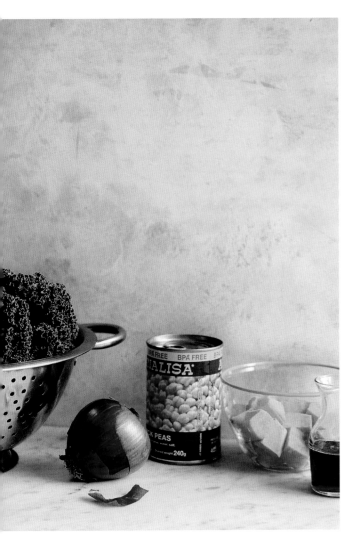
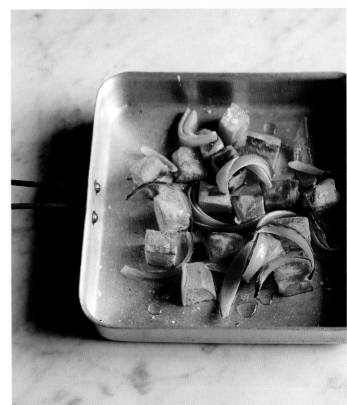
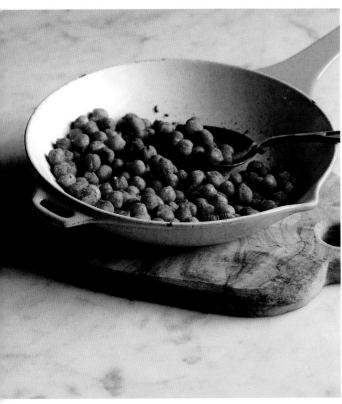
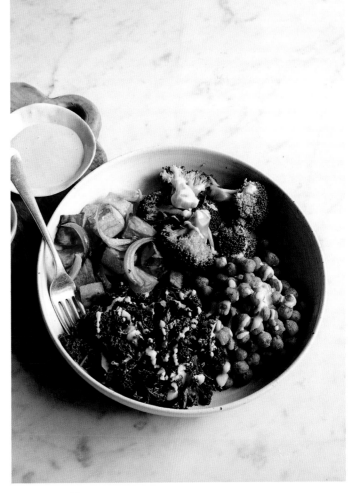

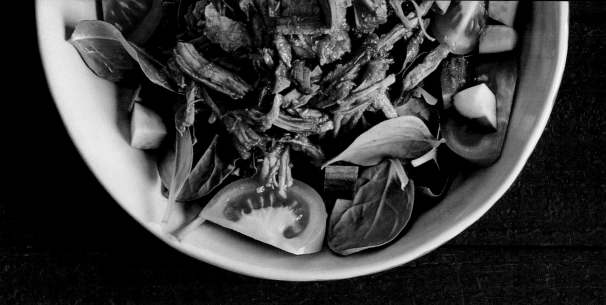

BULK COOK
USING RECIPE P. 38

ZESTY GREEK SALAD WITH PULLED PORK

SERVES
5

PREPARATION
10 MINS

COOK
5 MINS, PLUS
BASE RECIPE

COST PER SERVE
$1.90

1 x quantity Pulled Pork
(see p. 38)
¾ cup reduced-fat plain
Greek yoghurt
2 garlic cloves, crushed
2 tablespoons lemon juice
salt and freshly ground
black pepper
120 g baby spinach leaves
3 tomatoes, cut into wedges
2 Lebanese cucumbers, diced

Reheat the pulled pork in the microwave or on the stovetop until warmed through.

Combine the yoghurt, garlic and lemon juice in a bowl and season with salt and pepper.

Toss together the baby spinach, tomato and cucumber in a bowl.

Divide the salad evenly among five bowls and top with the pulled pork. Dollop with the yoghurt sauce and serve.

Store any leftover pulled pork in an airtight container in the fridge for 3–4 days or freeze for up to 3 months.

NUTRI DETAILS PER SERVE

1362 kJ/324 cals	Sat fat: 4.7 g
Protein: 29.9 g	Carbs: 13 g
Fibre: 5.5 g	Total sugar: 12 g
Total fat: 15.5 g	Free sugar: 3.3 g

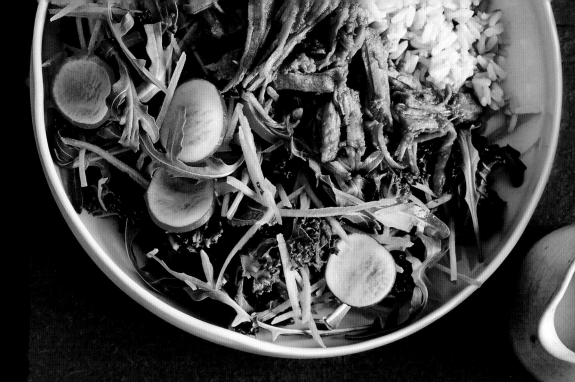

PULLED PORK, RICE AND KALE SALAD

BULK COOK
USING RECIPE P. 38

SERVES
5

PREPARATION
10 MINS

COOK
25 MINS, PLUS BASE RECIPE

COST PER SERVE
$1.21

¾ cup brown rice
1 x quantity Pulled Pork
  (see p. 38)
120 g kale leaves, chopped
60 g rocket leaves
2 radishes, sliced
½ carrot, grated
2 tablespoons lemon juice
1¼ tablespoons extra-virgin
  olive oil

NUTRI DETAILS PER SERVE

1304 kJ/310 cals	Sat fat: 2.9 g
Protein: 22.4 g	Carbs: 25.4 g
Fibre: 7.3 g	Total sugar: 6 g
Total fat: 11.8 g	Free sugar: 2 g

Bring 3 cups of water to the boil in a medium saucepan, add the rice and simmer for 25 minutes until tender. Drain. You could use pre-cooked rice for this recipe if you have some on hand. Just warm it through first.

Meanwhile, reheat the pulled pork in the microwave or on the stovetop until warmed through.

Combine the kale, rocket, radish and carrot in a bowl. Dress with the lemon juice and olive oil and gently toss to coat.

Divide the rice and pulled pork evenly among five bowls. Top with the kale salad and serve.

Store any leftover pulled pork in an airtight container in the fridge for 3–4 days or freeze for up to 3 months.

POTATO SALAD WITH SPINACH AND CHORIZO

SERVES
1

PREPARATION
10 MINS

COOK
10 MINS

COST PER SERVE
$2.45

---

1 potato (about 120 g),
   cut into bite-sized pieces
40 g chorizo sausage, sliced
2 tablespoons reduced-fat
   plain Greek yoghurt
1 tablespoon reduced-fat
   mayonnaise
1 tablespoon chopped
   flat-leaf parsley leaves
1 tablespoon lemon juice
30 g baby spinach leaves
1 hard-boiled free-range egg,
   peeled and quartered
1 tablespoon grated
   parmesan

NUTRI DETAILS PER SERVE

1680 kJ/400 cals	Sat fat: 6.9 g
Protein: 26.8 g	Carbs: 28.3 g
Fibre: 8.4 g	Total sugar: 13.9 g
Total fat: 17.7 g	Free sugar: 0 g

Steam the potato in the microwave or on the stovetop until tender. Set aside to cool.

Meanwhile, heat a frying pan over medium–high heat. Add the chorizo and cook for 2–3 minutes on each side until golden and crisp.

Place the yoghurt, mayonnaise, parsley and lemon juice in a bowl and mix well to make a dressing.

Combine the potato, chorizo, baby spinach and egg in a bowl. Drizzle over the dressing and gently toss to combine. Sprinkle with the parmesan and serve.

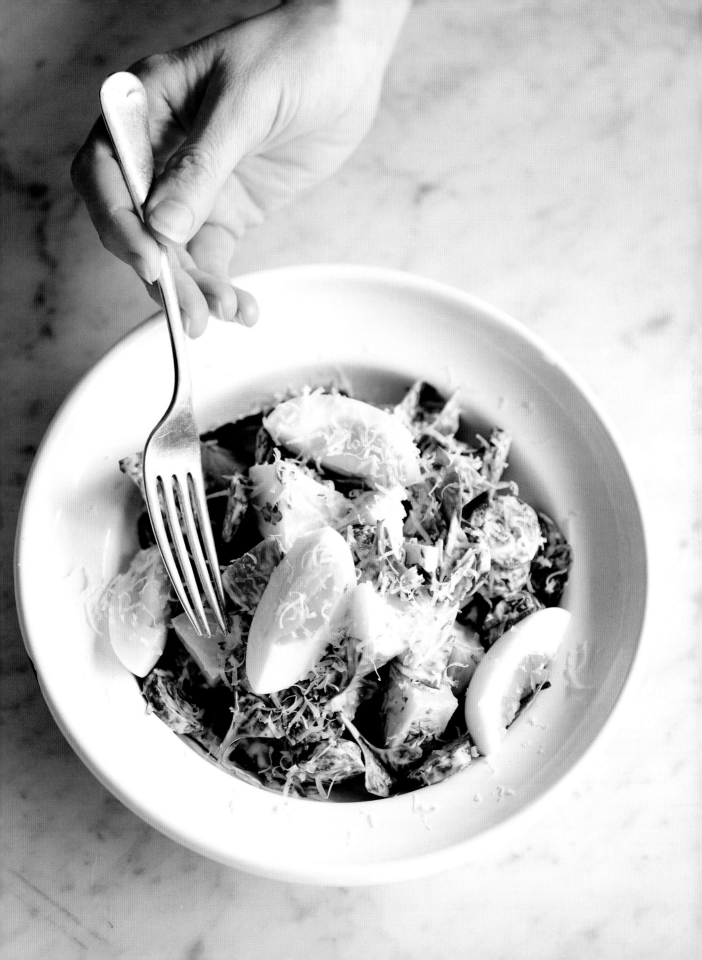

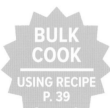

BULK COOK

USING RECIPE
P. 39

CAJUN CHICKEN SALAD BOWL

SERVES
6

PREPARATION
10 MINS

COOK
25 MINS, PLUS
BASE RECIPE

COST PER SERVE
$2.50

---

2 small sweet potatoes,
 peeled and diced
3 carrots, chopped
cooking oil spray
salt and freshly ground
 black pepper
1½ cups quinoa, rinsed
1 x quantity Cajun Chicken
 (see p. 39)
180 g kale leaves, chopped
180 g baby spinach leaves
¼ cup lemon juice

NUTRI DETAILS PER SERVE

1742 kJ/415 cals	Sat fat: 1.7 g
Protein: 31.7 g	Carbs: 51 g
Fibre: 11.8 g	Total sugar: 11.2 g
Total fat: 7.8 g	Free sugar: 0 g

Preheat the oven to 180°C and line a baking tray with baking paper.

Spread the sweet potato and carrot over the prepared tray in a single layer and lightly spray with cooking oil. Season with salt and pepper and roast for 20–25 minutes until tender.

Meanwhile, place the quinoa and 3 cups of water in a medium saucepan and bring to the boil. Reduce the heat and simmer, covered, for 15 minutes until tender and most of the liquid has been absorbed. Fluff up with a fork, then set aside to cool.

Reheat the Cajun chicken in the microwave or on the stovetop until warmed through.

Combine the kale, baby spinach, quinoa and roasted sweet potato and carrot in a large bowl and drizzle with the lemon juice.

Divide the salad among six bowls, top with the Cajun chicken and serve.

Store any leftovers in an airtight container in the fridge for 3–4 days. Leftover Cajun chicken can be stored in an airtight container in the fridge for 3–4 days or frozen for up to 2 months.

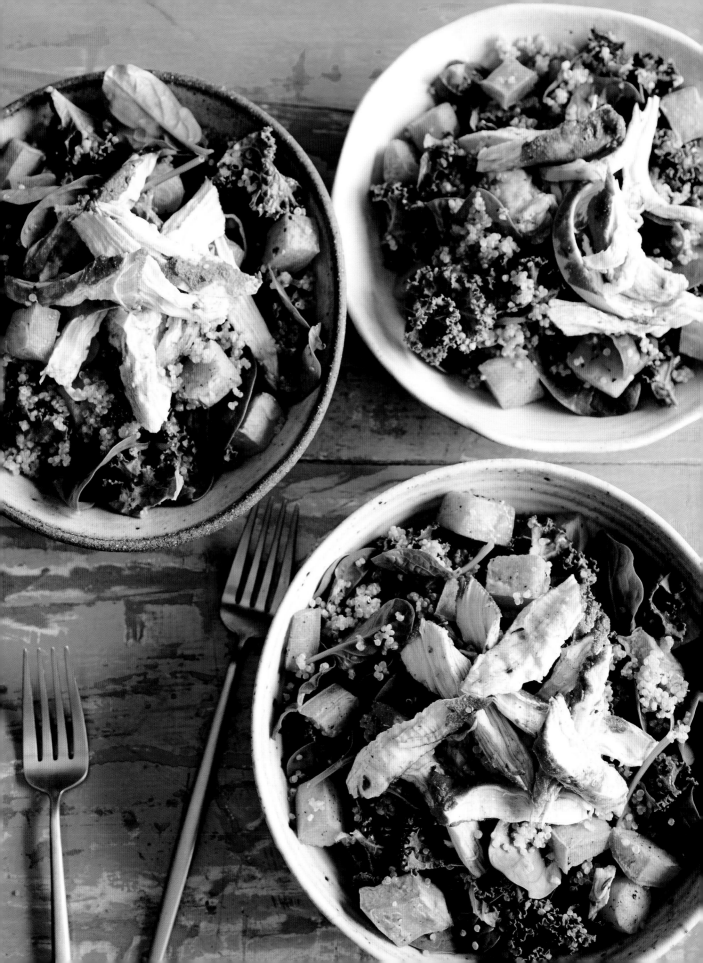

GREEK TUNA SALAD

SERVES
1

PREPARATION
10 MINS

COST PER SERVE
$1.50

---

1 x 95 g can tuna in spring
    water, drained
¼ Lebanese cucumber,
    chopped
½ red capsicum, diced
¼ red onion, diced
½ tomato, chopped
6 pitted kalamata olives,
    chopped
2 teaspoons red wine vinegar
1 teaspoon extra-virgin
    olive oil
¼ teaspoon dried oregano

Combine the tuna, cucumber, capsicum, onion, tomato and olives in a bowl.

Whisk the vinegar, olive oil and dried oregano in a bowl to make a dressing. Drizzle over the salad, toss to combine and serve.

NUTRI DETAILS PER SERVE

839 kJ/199 cals
Protein: 20.5 g
Fibre: 2.9 g
Total fat: 8.6 g

Sat fat: 1.8 g
Carbs: 8.8 g
Total sugar: 8.2 g
Free sugar: 0 g

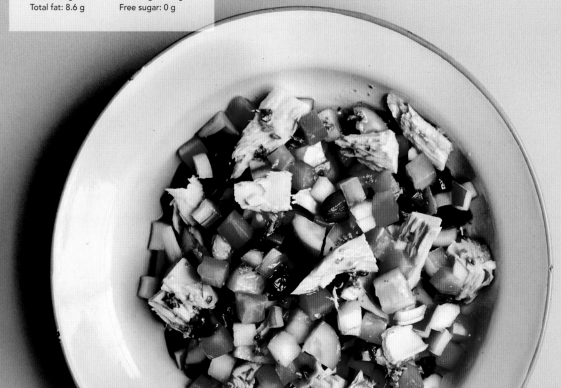

BACON PASTA SALAD

SERVES
1

PREPARATION
10 MINS

COOK
10 MINS

COST PER SERVE
$0.90

- 50 g wholemeal pasta
- 1 lean bacon rasher, trimmed and chopped
- 1 tablespoon reduced-fat ricotta
- 1 tablespoon reduced-fat mayonnaise
- ¼ cup shredded white cabbage
- ¼ cup shredded red cabbage
- 1 spring onion, sliced
- ¼ red capsicum, finely sliced
- ½ carrot, grated

NUTRI DETAILS PER SERVE

1294 kJ/309 cals	Sat fat: 1.3 g
Protein: 17.3 g	Carbs: 43.4 g
Fibre: 8.2 g	Total sugar: 8.6 g
Total fat: 5.1 g	Free sugar: 0 g

Cook the pasta in a saucepan of boiling water according to packet directions. Drain.

Meanwhile, place the bacon in a frying pan over medium–high heat and cook until crisp. Drain on paper towel and set aside to cool.

Combine the ricotta and mayonnaise in a bowl.

Place the white and red cabbage, spring onion, capsicum and carrot in a large bowl. Add the cooked pasta, bacon and ricotta dressing, gently toss to combine and serve.

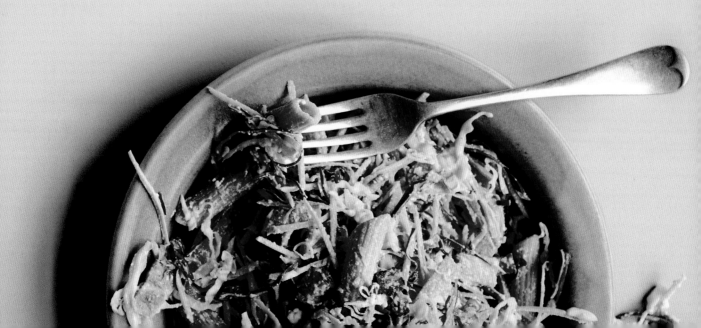

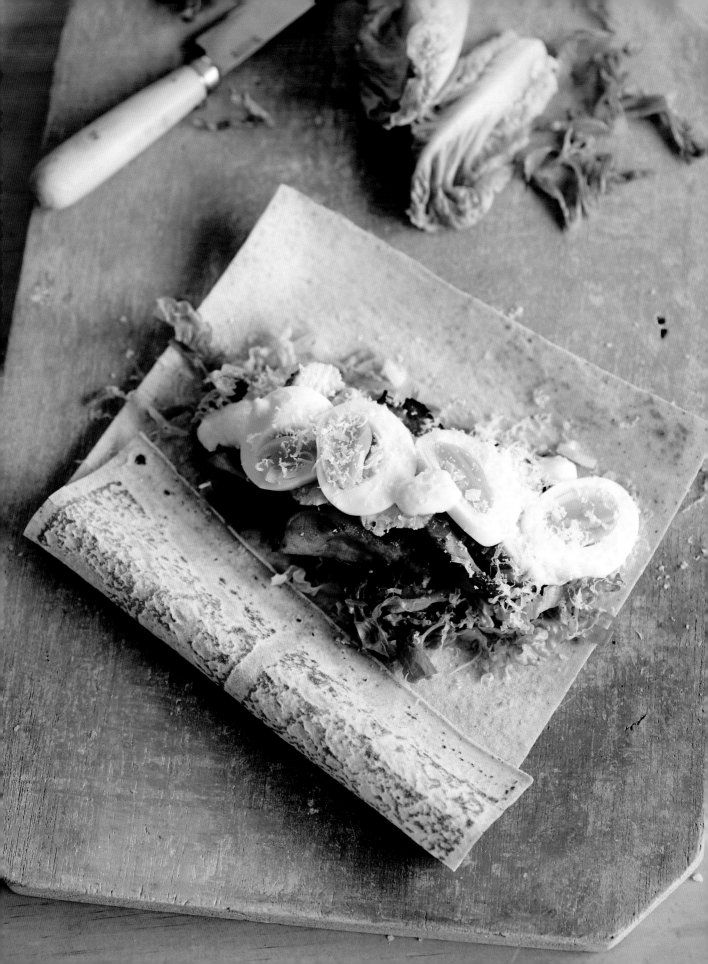

CHICKEN CAESAR WRAP

SERVES
1

PREPARATION
10 MINS

COOK
6 MINS

COST PER SERVE
$2.00

1 teaspoon extra-virgin olive oil
40 g chicken breast fillet
1 slice lean smoked ham, sliced
1 tablespoon reduced-fat plain Greek yoghurt
2 teaspoons lemon juice
1 wholemeal mountain bread wrap
½ cup shredded cos lettuce
1 hard-boiled free-range egg, peeled and sliced
1 tablespoon grated parmesan

NUTRI DETAILS PER SERVE

1289 kJ/307 cals
Protein: 25.4 g
Fibre: 1.8 g
Total fat: 15.8 g

Sat fat: 5 g
Carbs: 14.7 g
Total sugar: 3.7 g
Free sugar: 0 g

Heat the olive oil in a non-stick frying pan over medium–high heat. Add the chicken and cook for 2–3 minutes on each side until golden and cooked through.

Shortly before the chicken is ready, add the ham to the pan and cook for 1–2 minutes until slightly crisp. Set the chicken and ham aside to cool, then slice the chicken.

Whisk the yoghurt and lemon juice in a bowl to make a dressing.

Top the wrap with the shredded lettuce, chicken, ham and egg. Sprinkle with the grated parmesan and drizzle over the dressing. Roll up the wrap and enjoy.

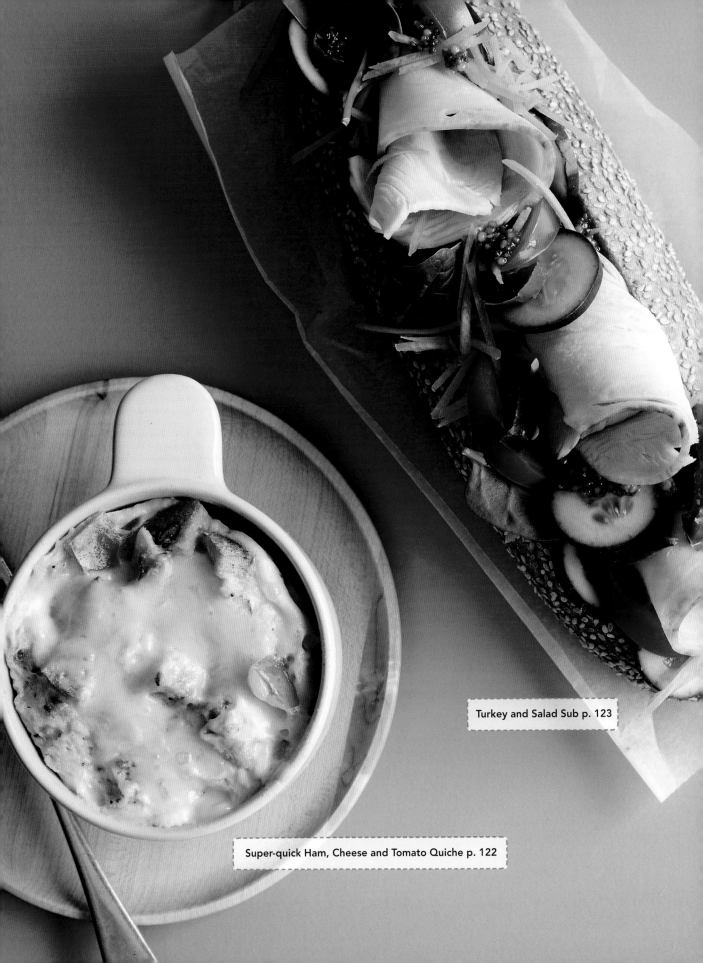

Turkey and Salad Sub p. 123

Super-quick Ham, Cheese and Tomato Quiche p. 122

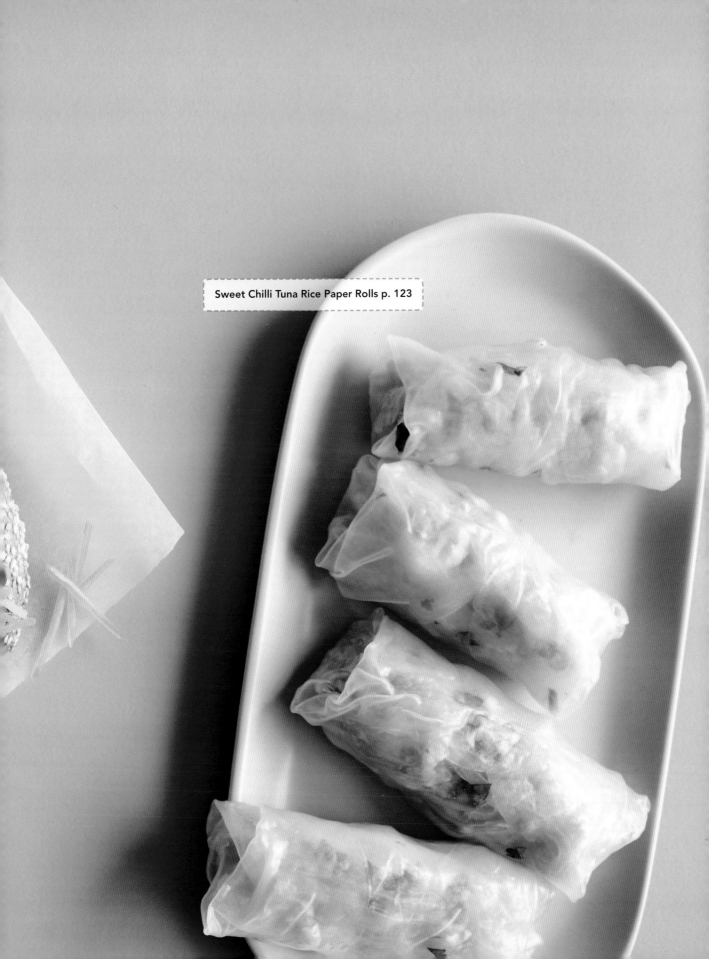

Sweet Chilli Tuna Rice Paper Rolls p. 123

SUPER-QUICK HAM, CHEESE AND TOMATO QUICHE

SERVES
1

PREPARATION
5 MINS

COOK
2 MINS

COST PER SERVE
$1.75

½ teaspoon butter, melted
2 free-range eggs
2 tablespoons reduced-fat milk of choice
1 slice lean smoked ham, diced
1 tablespoon light cream cheese
½ tomato, chopped
½ slice wholegrain or gluten-free bread of choice, cut into bite-sized cubes
2 teaspoons grated reduced-fat cheddar

NUTRI DETAILS PER SERVE

1308 kJ/311 cals	Sat fat: 7.7 g
Protein: 25 g	Carbs: 11.5 g
Fibre: 1.8 g	Total sugar: 4.4 g
Total fat: 18 g	Free sugar: 0 g

Place the melted butter, eggs and milk in a 250 ml mug or ramekin and whisk to combine.

Add the ham, cream cheese, tomato and bread cubes and stir to combine. Top with the cheddar and microwave on high for 90 seconds. If the egg is not set after this time, microwave for an additional 30 seconds or until cooked through.

Allow to cool slightly and serve.

TURKEY AND SALAD SUB

SERVES
1

PREPARATION
10 MINS

COST PER SERVE
$2.50

½ teaspoon honey
1 teaspoon wholegrain mustard
1 wholegrain long roll
3 slices lean smoked turkey
½ carrot, grated
handful of baby spinach leaves
¼ tomato, sliced
¼ Lebanese cucumber, sliced
1 teaspoon sliced pickled jalapeno chilli

Combine the honey and mustard in a small bowl.

Slice the bread roll in half and spread the bottom half with the honey–mustard mixture.

Top with the turkey, carrot, spinach, tomato, cucumber and chilli. Sandwich with the other half of the roll and serve.

NUTRI DETAILS PER SERVE

1474 kJ/351 cals	Sat fat: 0.9 g
Protein: 27.3 g	Carbs: 44 g
Fibre: 7.3 g	Total sugar: 9.2 g
Total fat: 5.5 g	Free sugar: 2.9 g

SWEET CHILLI TUNA RICE PAPER ROLLS

SERVES
1

PREPARATION
10 MINS

COST PER SERVE
$2.22

1 x 185 g can tuna in spring water, drained
1 tablespoon sweet chilli sauce
4 rice paper sheets
1 carrot, grated
1 cup bean sprouts, trimmed
1 tablespoon chopped coriander leaves

Combine the tuna and half the sweet chilli sauce in a bowl.

Lay a damp tea towel on a workbench and fill a wide shallow bowl with cold water.

Place one rice paper sheet in the water for about 5 seconds to soften. Carefully remove it from the water and lay it flat on the damp tea towel.

Arrange one-quarter of the carrot, bean sprouts, tuna mixture and coriander in the centre of the sheet. Fold the top and bottom into the centre, then roll up to enclose the filling.

Repeat with the remaining ingredients to make four rolls. Serve with the remaining sweet chilli sauce for dipping.

NUTRI DETAILS PER SERVE

1528 kJ/363 cals	Sat fat: 1.7 g
Protein: 47.3 g	Carbs: 30.4 g
Fibre: 3.7 g	Total sugar: 14.9 g
Total fat: 5.1 g	Free sugar: 10 g

SOUPS

Batch cook for easy meals!

SLOW-COOKED VEGETABLE AND TORTELLINI SOUP

SERVES
9

PREPARATION
15 MINS

COOK
40 MINS (8 HOURS IN A SLOW COOKER)

COST PER SERVE
$1.74

2 tablespoons extra-virgin olive oil
1 brown onion, diced
120 g pumpkin, peeled and seeds removed, diced
2 carrots, diced
2 celery stalks, diced
1 tablespoon tomato paste
3 garlic cloves, grated
2 litres salt-reduced vegetable stock
1 × 400 g can diced tomatoes
2 teaspoons dried Italian herbs
1 tablespoon chopped flat-leaf parsley leaves
salt and freshly ground black pepper
1 × 400 g can cannellini beans, drained and rinsed
1 × 400 g can kidney beans, drained and rinsed
120 g green beans, trimmed and chopped
2 small zucchini, diced
400 g fresh spinach and ricotta tortellini
60 g baby spinach leaves
¼ cup grated parmesan

NUTRI DETAILS PER SERVE

1366 kJ/326 cals
Protein: 14.9 g
Fibre: 11 g
Total fat: 7.9 g
Sat fat: 1.9 g
Carbs: 41.8 g
Total sugar: 6.4 g
Free sugar: 0.2 g

If cooking on the stovetop:

Heat the olive oil in a large saucepan over medium–high heat. Add the onion, pumpkin, carrot and celery and cook for 4–5 minutes until the onion is translucent.

Add the tomato paste and garlic and cook for 1 minute, then stir in the stock and canned tomatoes. Add the dried herbs and parsley and season to taste with salt and pepper. Bring to the boil, then reduce the heat and simmer, covered, for 20–25 minutes, stirring occasionally.

Add the cannellini and kidney beans, green beans, zucchini and tortellini. Cook for 5 minutes until the vegetables are tender and the pasta is al dente. Pour in 1–2 cups of water if the soup becomes too thick.

Stir through the spinach, cover and cook for a further 2 minutes until wilted.

If cooking in a slow cooker:

Place the onion, pumpkin, carrot, celery, tomato paste, garlic, stock, canned tomatoes, dried herbs and parsley in the slow cooker dish. Season with salt and pepper and mix well to combine. Cover and cook on low heat for 6–8 hours.

Add the cannellini and kidney beans, green beans, zucchini and tortellini and cook on high heat for another 30 minutes until the vegetables are tender and the pasta is al dente. Pour in 1–2 cups of water if the soup becomes too thick.

Stir through the spinach, cover and cook for a further 5 minutes until wilted.

To serve:

Divide the soup evenly among bowls and top with a sprinkling of grated parmesan.

Store any leftover soup in an airtight container in the fridge for 4–5 days or freeze in portions for up to 4 months.

SUITABLE TO FREEZE

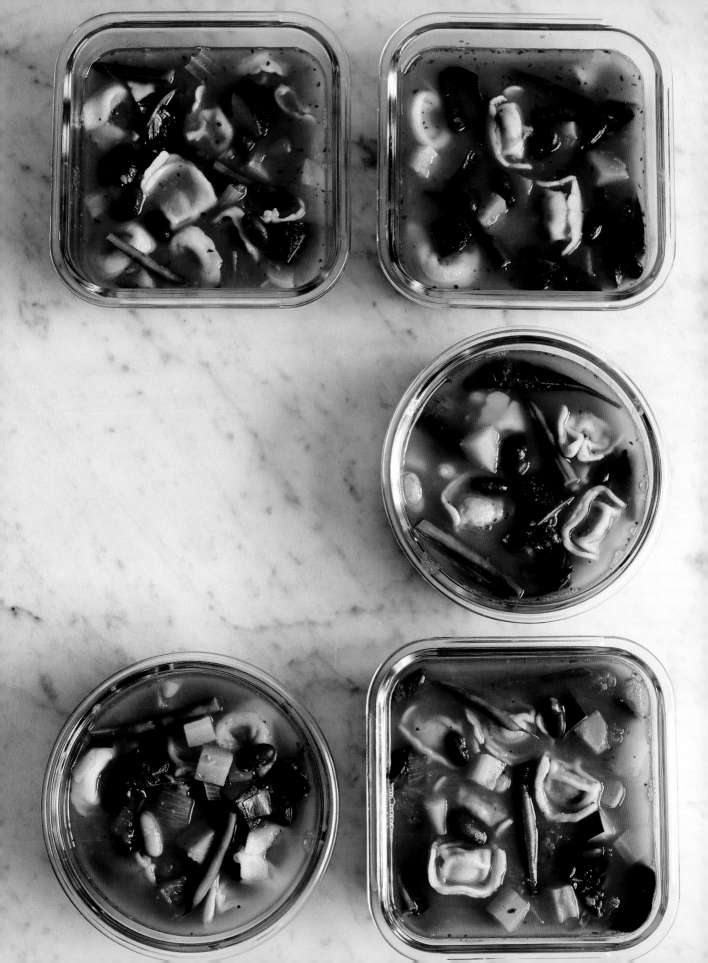

COCONUTTY PUMPKIN SOUP

SERVES
4

PREPARATION
15 MINS

COOK
20 MINS

COST PER SERVE
$2.20

2 tablespoons extra-virgin olive oil
2 brown onions, diced
4 celery stalks, diced
4 carrots, chopped
1 teaspoon ground cumin
1 teaspoon ground coriander
1 teaspoon chilli powder
1 teaspoon ground turmeric
960 g pumpkin, peeled and seeds removed, chopped
2 litres salt-reduced vegetable stock
salt and freshly ground black pepper
⅔ cup coconut cream
½ cup coriander leaves

Heat the olive oil in a large saucepan over medium heat, add the onion, celery and carrot and cook for 5 minutes until starting to soften. Add the ground spices and stir for a few minutes until fragrant, then add the pumpkin and stir to combine.

Pour in the stock. Bring to the boil, then reduce the heat and simmer for 10 minutes until the vegetables are soft.

Using a benchtop or stick blender, blitz the soup until smooth, adding a little water if the consistency is too thick. Season to taste with salt and pepper.

Divide the soup among four bowls. Drizzle over the coconut cream and finish with a sprinkling of coriander.

Store any leftovers in an airtight container in the fridge for 3–4 days or freeze in portions for up to 3 months.

SUITABLE TO FREEZE

NUTRI DETAILS PER SERVE

1178 kJ/280 cals	Sat fat: 9.4 g
Protein: 8.8 g	Carbs: 15.4 g
Fibre: 5.6 g	Total sugar: 10 g
Total fat: 19.4 g	Free sugar: 0 g

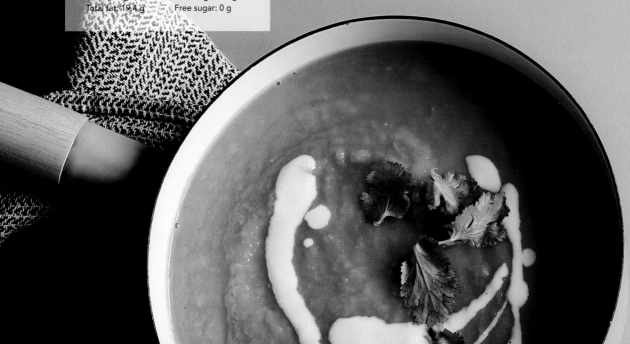

SPICY CHICKEN AND CORN SOUP

SERVES
4

PREPARATION
10 MINS

COOK
15 MINS

COST PER SERVE
$2.47

1 tablespoon coconut oil
2 cups corn kernels (fresh or canned)
1 teaspoon dried chilli flakes
1 tablespoon grated ginger
4 spring onions, finely sliced
2 litres salt-reduced chicken stock
360 g chicken breast fillets
4 free-range eggs, lightly beaten
1 tablespoon tamari (gluten-free soy sauce)

NUTRI DETAILS PER SERVE

1597 kJ/380 cals
Protein: 34.2 g
Fibre: 2.8 g
Total fat: 17.8 g

Sat fat: 8.8 g
Carbs: 19.4 g
Total sugar: 4.2 g
Free sugar: 0 g

Heat the coconut oil in a saucepan over medium–high heat, add the corn and cook for 1–2 minutes. Add the chilli flakes, ginger and half the spring onion and stir until fragrant.

Pour in the stock and bring to the boil. Add the chicken, then reduce the heat and simmer, covered, for 10 minutes until the chicken is cooked through.

Using tongs, remove the chicken from the soup and shred with two forks. Return the chicken to the soup.

Gradually stir the egg into the simmering soup to cook through, then stir through the tamari.

Divide the soup among four bowls, top with the remaining spring onion and serve.

Store any leftovers in an airtight container in the fridge for 3–4 days or freeze in portions for up to 3 months.

SUITABLE TO FREEZE

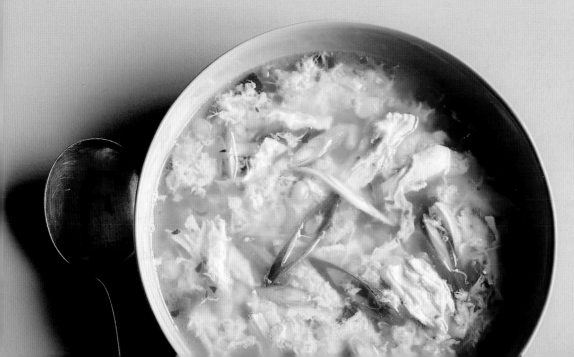

BEEF, LENTIL AND VEGGIE SOUP

SERVES
4

PREPARATION
10 MINS, PLUS
SOAKING TIME

COOK
1 HOUR
45 MINS

COST PER SERVE
$1.89

¾ cup dried brown lentils
1 tablespoon extra-virgin
  olive oil
400 g stewing steak (such as
  lean chuck steak), trimmed
  and cut into 2 cm cubes
1 potato, diced
2 carrots, diced
1 teaspoon curry powder
1 litre salt-reduced beef
  stock, plus extra if needed
½ cup corn kernels (fresh
  or canned)
½ cup frozen peas
200 ml reduced-fat
  coconut milk
salt and freshly ground
  black pepper
flat-leaf parsley leaves,
  to serve (optional)

NUTRI DETAILS PER SERVE

1628 kJ/387 cals	Sat fat: 6 g
Protein: 34.6 g	Carbs: 26.8 g
Fibre: 8.7 g	Total sugar: 4.3 g
Total fat: 14 g	Free sugar: 0 g

Place the lentils in a bowl, cover with water and leave to soak overnight. Drain and rinse two or three times to make sure you remove any impurities in the bowl.

Heat the olive oil in a large saucepan or flameproof casserole dish over medium–high heat. Add the beef and cook for 4–5 minutes until browned all over.

Add the drained lentils, potato, carrot, curry powder and stock and stir to combine well. Bring to the boil, then reduce the heat to medium–low and simmer, covered, for 1–1½ hours until the meat is really tender and falling apart. Add some extra stock or water if the soup becomes too thick.

About 10 minutes before you are ready to serve, stir in the corn, peas and coconut milk and simmer until heated through.

Divide the soup among four bowls and season to taste with salt and pepper. Finish with a sprinkling of fresh parsley leaves, if you like.

Store any leftovers in an airtight container in the fridge for 3–4 days or freeze in portions for up to 3 months.

SUITABLE TO FREEZE

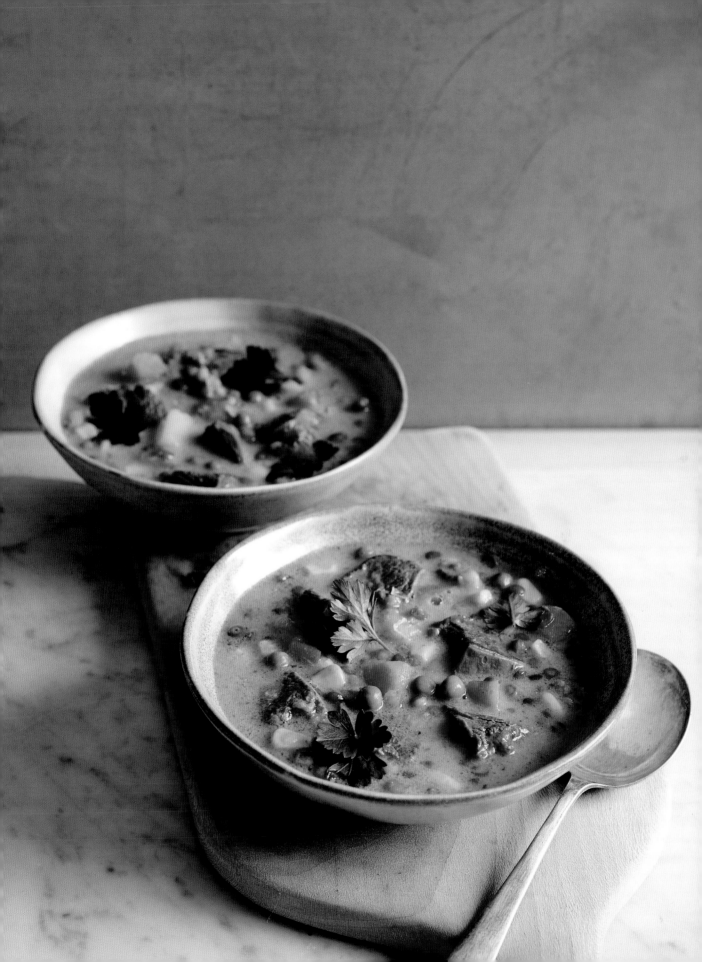

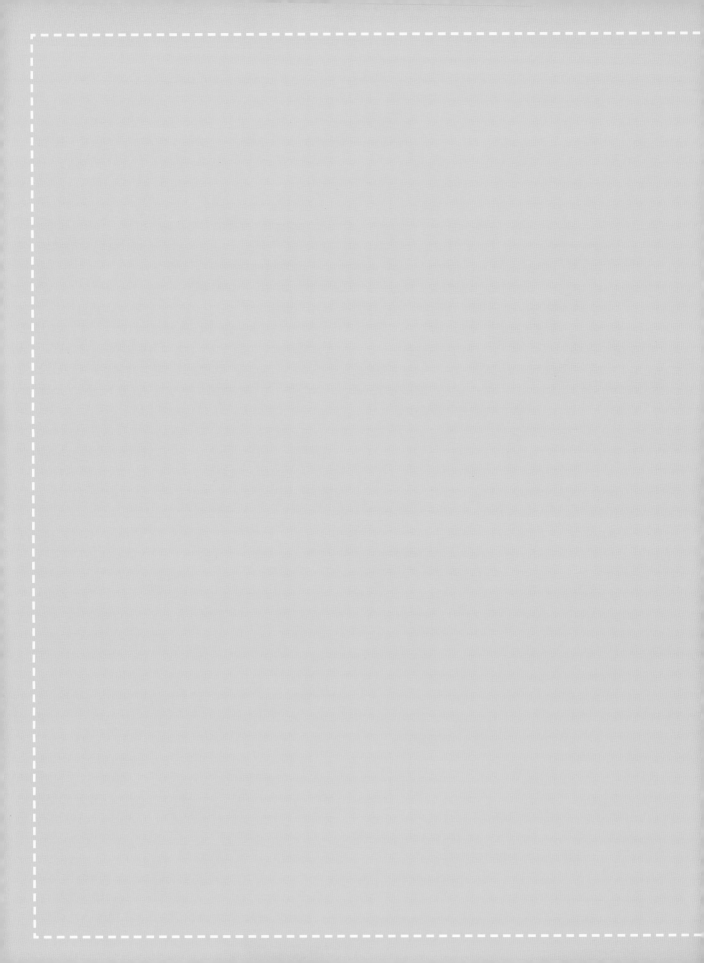

PASTA, NOODLES & RICE

Comfort without the calories!

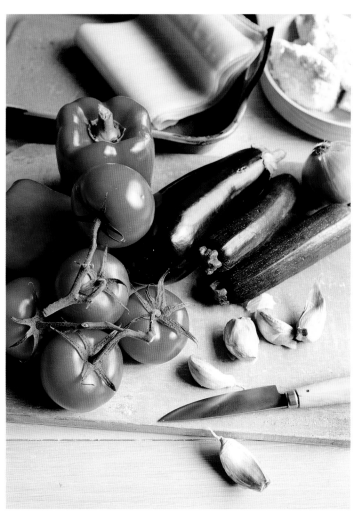

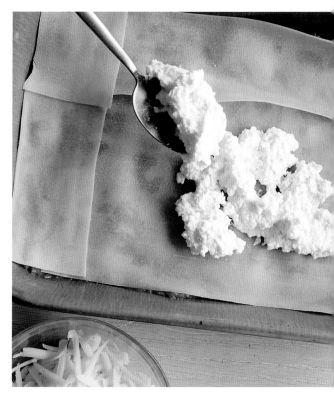

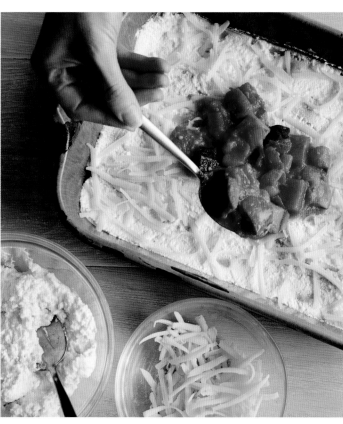

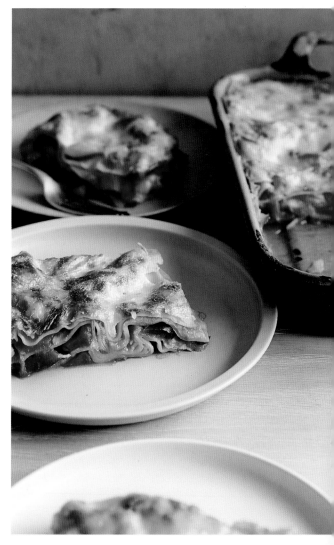

RATATOUILLE LASAGNE

SERVES
8

PREPARATION
15 MINS

COOK
1 HOUR 15 MINS

COST PER SERVE
$1.78

1 tablespoon extra-virgin olive oil
2 garlic cloves, grated
1 brown onion, diced
1 small zucchini, diced
2 red capsicums, diced
½ eggplant, diced
8 tomatoes, diced
2 tablespoons tomato paste
cooking oil spray
10 fresh lasagne sheets
400 g reduced-fat ricotta
1 cup grated reduced-fat cheddar

NUTRI DETAILS PER SERVE

1370 kJ/326 cals	Sat fat: 3.9 g
Protein: 18 g	Carbs: 43 g
Fibre: 5.8 g	Total sugar: 8.4 g
Total fat: 7 g	Free sugar: 0 g

Heat the olive oil in a frying pan over medium–high heat, add the garlic and onion and cook for 1–2 minutes until the onion is translucent. Stir in the zucchini, capsicum, eggplant and tomato.

Add the tomato paste and 2 cups of water and stir to combine. Bring to the boil, then reduce the heat and simmer for 25 minutes until the vegetables are very tender and the sauce has thickened.

Preheat the oven to 200°C and lightly spray a large baking dish with cooking oil.

Spread one-third of the sauce over the base of the prepared dish and top with a layer of lasagne sheets. Spread with one-third of the ricotta, then sprinkle over one-third of the grated cheddar.

Repeat with the remaining sauce, lasagne sheets, ricotta and grated cheese to make three layers in all, finishing with a top layer of grated cheddar.

Cover the dish with foil and bake for 30 minutes. Remove the foil and bake for another 15 minutes until the cheese is melted and golden.

Allow the lasagne to sit for a few minutes before cutting into eight portions. One portion is one serve. Serve as is or with a simple salad, if you like.

Store any leftovers in an airtight container in the fridge for 3–4 days or freeze for up to 3 months.

SUITABLE TO FREEZE

SAUSAGE AND VEGETABLE PASTA BAKE

SERVES	PREPARATION	COOK	COST PER SERVE
4	15 MINS	35 MINS	$1.55

200 g wholemeal pasta
(any shape)
1 tablespoon extra-virgin
olive oil
2 garlic cloves, chopped
1 brown onion, chopped
280 g lean sausages of
choice, sliced
2 carrots, grated
1 small zucchini, grated
120 g pumpkin, peeled and
seeds removed, grated
2 tablespoons tomato paste
1 × 400 g can diced tomatoes
salt and freshly ground
black pepper
½ cup grated reduced-fat
cheddar

NUTRI DETAILS PER SERVE

1903 kJ/455 cals	Sat fat: 8.4 g
Protein: 26.7 g	Carbs: 37.1 g
Fibre: 8.4 g	Total sugar: 9.9 g
Total fat: 20.1 g	Free sugar: 0 g

Preheat the oven to 180°C.

Cook the pasta in a saucepan of boiling water according to packet directions. Drain.

Meanwhile, heat the olive oil in a large frying pan over medium–low heat. Add the garlic and onion and cook for 2 minutes, then add the sausage pieces and cook for 5 minutes until nicely browned.

Add the carrot, zucchini, pumpkin and ¼ cup of water. Simmer, stirring gently, for 2 minutes until the vegetables begin to soften. Mix through the tomato paste and canned tomatoes, season to taste with salt and pepper and simmer for a further 5 minutes.

Remove the pan from the heat and stir in the drained pasta. Transfer the mixture to a large baking dish and sprinkle the cheese over the top. Bake for 20 minutes until the cheese is melted and golden. Allow to cool slightly, then divide equally among four plates and serve.

Store any leftovers in an airtight container in the fridge for 3–4 days or freeze for up to 3 months.

SUITABLE TO FREEZE

You could also spoon the pasta bake into smaller dishes or a silicone muffin tray for individual serves.

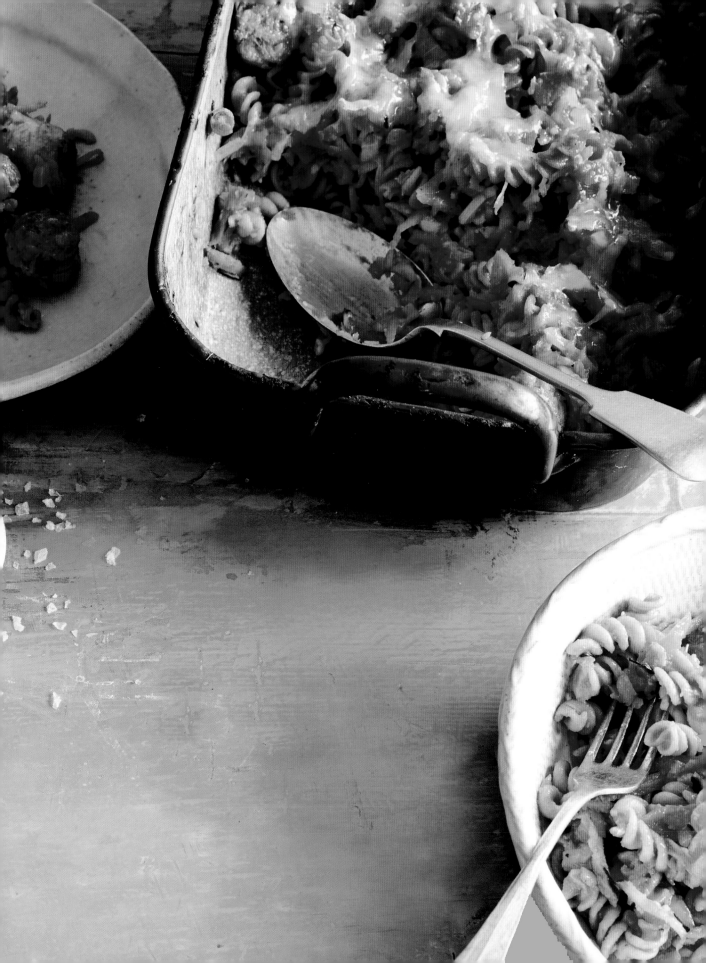

MEDITERRANEAN CHICKEN
AND VEGETABLE PASTA

SERVES
4

PREPARATION
10 MINS

COOK
15 MINS

COST PER SERVE
$2.50

160 g wholemeal pasta
(any shape)
1 tablespoon extra-virgin
olive oil
400 g chicken breast fillets
salt and freshly ground
black pepper
1 brown onion, diced
3 garlic cloves, crushed
1 eggplant, diced
2 small zucchini, diced
1 cup tomato passata
1 teaspoon dried chilli flakes
2 teaspoons dried Italian
herbs
⅓ cup basil leaves

NUTRI DETAILS PER SERVE

1570 kJ/374 cals	Sat fat: 2.5 g
Protein: 30 g	Carbs: 33 g
Fibre: 9.3 g	Total sugar: 7.9 g
Total fat: 11.6 g	Free sugar: 0 g

Cook the pasta in a saucepan of boiling water according to packet directions. Drain.

Meanwhile, heat the olive oil in a frying pan over medium–high heat. Season the chicken with salt and pepper, then add to the pan and cook for 4–5 minutes on each side until cooked through. Remove from the pan and set aside to rest.

Add the onion, garlic, eggplant and zucchini to the pan and cook for 4–5 minutes until tender. Stir in the passata, chilli flakes, dried herbs and most of the basil leaves and season to taste with salt and pepper.

Slice the chicken and add to the vegetable sauce, along with the drained pasta. Toss well to combine and serve scattered with the remaining basil leaves.

Store any leftovers in an airtight container in the fridge for 3–4 days or freeze for up to 3 months.

SUITABLE TO FREEZE

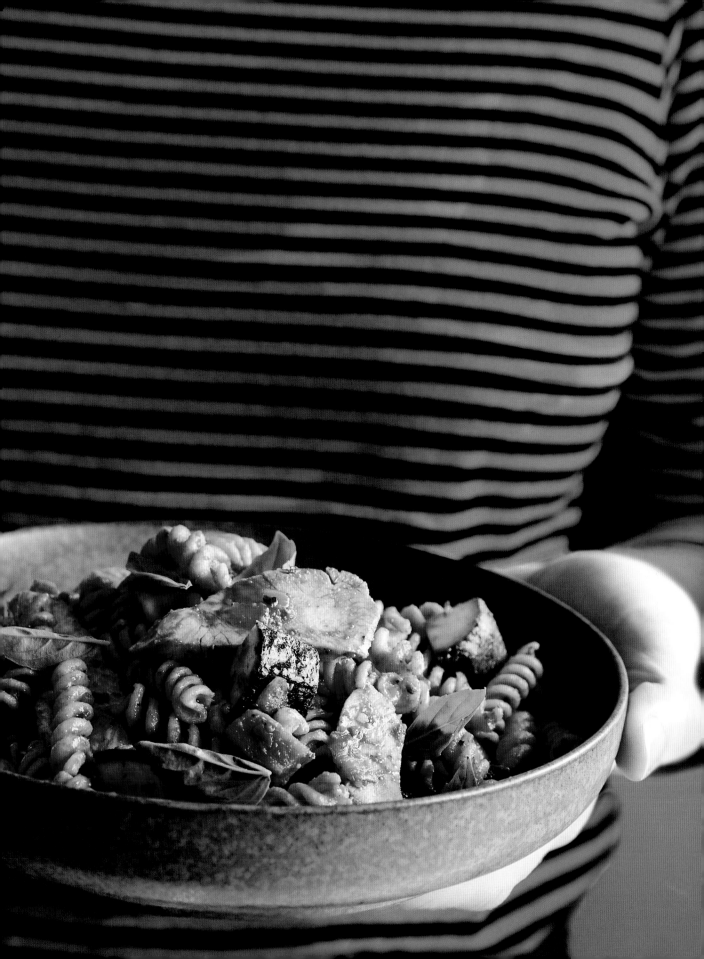

BAKED CHEESE AND TOMATO RISOTTO

SERVES
4

PREPARATION
10 MINS

COOK
1 HOUR

COST PER SERVE
$1.42

---

1 tablespoon extra-virgin
   olive oil
1 brown onion, finely diced
1 garlic clove, chopped
250 g cherry tomatoes
1 cup arborio rice
650 ml salt-reduced
   vegetable stock, plus extra
½ cup grated reduced-fat
   cheddar
2 teaspoons dried Italian herbs

NUTRI DETAILS PER SERVE

1280 kJ/306 cals	Sat fat: 3.8 g
Protein: 13.3 g	Carbs: 38.8 g
Fibre: 2.9 g	Total sugar: 2.6 g
Total fat: 9.8 g	Free sugar: 0 g

Preheat the oven to 200°C.

Combine the olive oil, onion, garlic and tomatoes in a baking dish. Bake for 15 minutes until the tomatoes are tender. Squash them gently with a fork to release the juices.

Add the rice to the dish and stir to coat in the tomato mixture. Pour over the stock, cover, then return to the oven and bake for 40–45 minutes until all the liquid has been absorbed and the rice is tender, removing the cover and stirring once halfway through, then replacing the cover.

Remove the dish from the oven. Stir through the grated cheese and sprinkle over the herbs. Stir through a little extra stock or water to loosen the risotto, if needed.

Serve with steamed vegetables or a side salad, if desired.

Store any leftover risotto in an airtight container in the fridge for 2–3 days or freeze for up to 3 months.

SUITABLE TO FREEZE

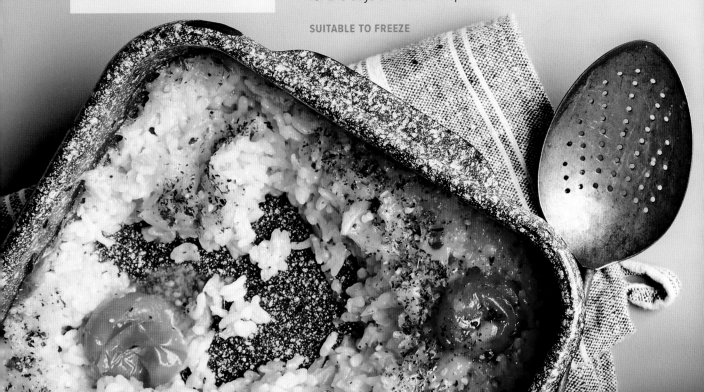

TUNA AND PUMPKIN MAC AND CHEESE

SERVES
4

PREPARATION
15 MINS

COOK
30 MINS

COST PER SERVE
$1.20

1 cup macaroni
480 g pumpkin, peeled and seeds removed, diced
salt and freshly ground black pepper
360 g drained canned tuna in spring water
4 garlic cloves, grated
1 tomato, sliced
½ cup grated reduced-fat cheddar

NUTRI DETAILS PER SERVE

1408 kJ/335 cals	Sat fat: 3.6 g
Protein: 34 g	Carbs: 30.3 g
Fibre: 5.8 g	Total sugar: 5.6 g
Total fat: 7.2 g	Free sugar: 0 g

Preheat the oven to 190°C.

Cook the macaroni in a saucepan of boiling water according to packet directions. Drain.

Meanwhile, steam the pumpkin in the microwave or on the stovetop for 10 minutes until very tender. Using a benchtop or stick blender, blitz until smooth. Season to taste with salt and pepper.

Combine the macaroni, pumpkin puree, tuna and garlic in a large baking dish. Top with tomato slices and sprinkle over the grated cheese. Bake for 20 minutes until the cheese is melted and golden.

Allow to cool slightly, then divide equally among four plates and serve.

Store any leftovers in an airtight container in the fridge for 3–4 days or freeze for up to 3 months.

SUITABLE TO FREEZE

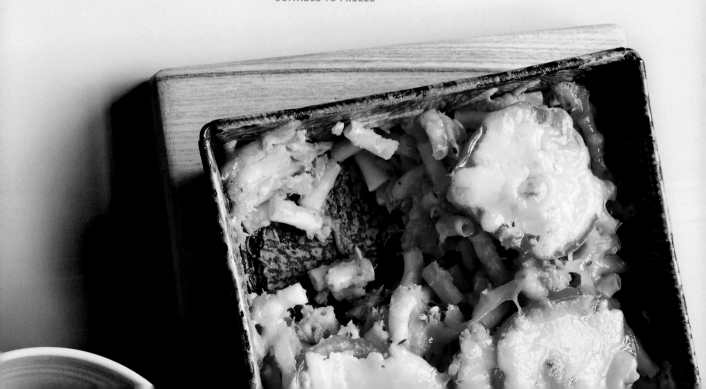

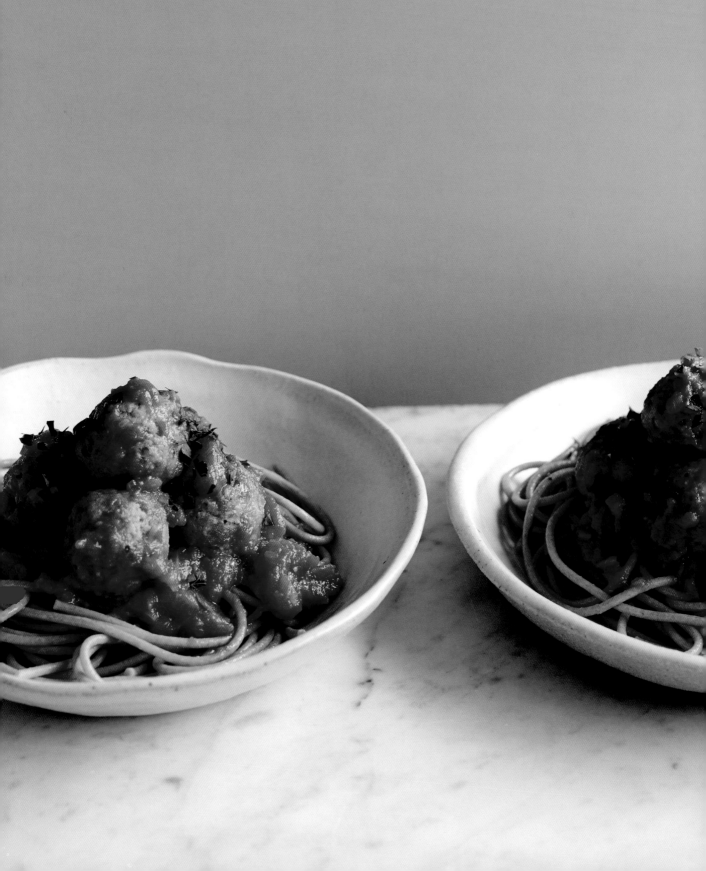

TURKEY MEATBALLS AND SPAGHETTI

SERVES
4

PREPARATION
15 MINS

COOK
40 MINS

COST PER SERVE
$2.15

400 g lean turkey mince
¼ cup dried wholemeal
    breadcrumbs
2½ teaspoons dried
    Italian herbs
1 free-range egg white
salt and freshly ground
    black pepper
2 teaspoons extra-virgin
    olive oil
1 brown onion, finely diced
2 garlic cloves, grated
800 g canned whole peeled
    tomatoes
⅓ cup tomato paste
boiling water, if needed
160 g wholemeal spaghetti
¼ cup flat-leaf parsley leaves,
    chopped

NUTRI DETAILS PER SERVE

1775 kJ/423 cals   Sat fat: 5.5 g
Protein: 27 g   Carbs: 36.3 g
Fibre: 8 g   Total sugar: 9.8 g
Total fat: 17.3 g   Free sugar: 0 g

Place the turkey mince, breadcrumbs, dried herbs and egg white in a bowl and season with salt and pepper. Mix together with a fork, then, using clean hands, form the mixture into 20–24 small meatballs.

Heat the olive oil in a non-stick frying pan with a lid over medium–high heat, add the meatballs and cook until browned on all sides. Remove from the pan and set aside.

Add the onion and garlic to the pan and cook for 1–2 minutes until softened. Add the canned tomatoes and tomato paste and season with salt and pepper. Stir well and bring to a simmer, breaking up the tomatoes with a wooden spoon if required.

Return the meatballs to the pan and pop the lid on. Reduce the heat to low and simmer for 20 minutes, adding a little boiling water if the sauce begins to look dry.

Meanwhile, cook the spaghetti in a large saucepan of boiling water according to packet directions.

Drain the spaghetti and divide among serving bowls. Top with the sauce and meatballs and garnish with the chopped parsley.

Store any leftovers in an airtight container in the fridge for 2–3 days or freeze for up to 3 months.

SUITABLE TO FREEZE

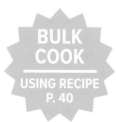

BULK COOK

USING RECIPE P. 40

ZOODLES WITH HIDDEN VEG BOLOGNESE

SERVES
4

PREPARATION
5 MINS

COOK
5 MINS, PLUS BASE RECIPE

COST PER SERVE
$1.92

---

1 x quantity Hidden Veg Bolognese (see p. 40)
4 small zucchini
2 tablespoons grated parmesan

NUTRI DETAILS PER SERVE

1013 kJ/241 cals	Sat fat: 4.2 g
Protein: 22 g	Carbs: 7.6 g
Fibre: 3.9 g	Total sugar: 6.3 g
Total fat: 12.8 g	Free sugar: 0 g

FOR A VEGETARIAN MEAL

Use vegetable stock and replace the mince in the sauce with 800 g canned lentils, drained and rinsed.

COST PER SERVE $1.70

Reheat the hidden veg bolognese in the microwave or on the stovetop until warmed through.

Meanwhile, use a spiraliser or peeler to slice the zucchini into noodles. Blanch in boiling water for 1 minute or less until just tender.

Top the zucchini noodles with bolognese and sprinkle with parmesan to serve.

Store any leftover bolognese in an airtight container in the fridge for 2–3 days or freeze for up to 3 months.

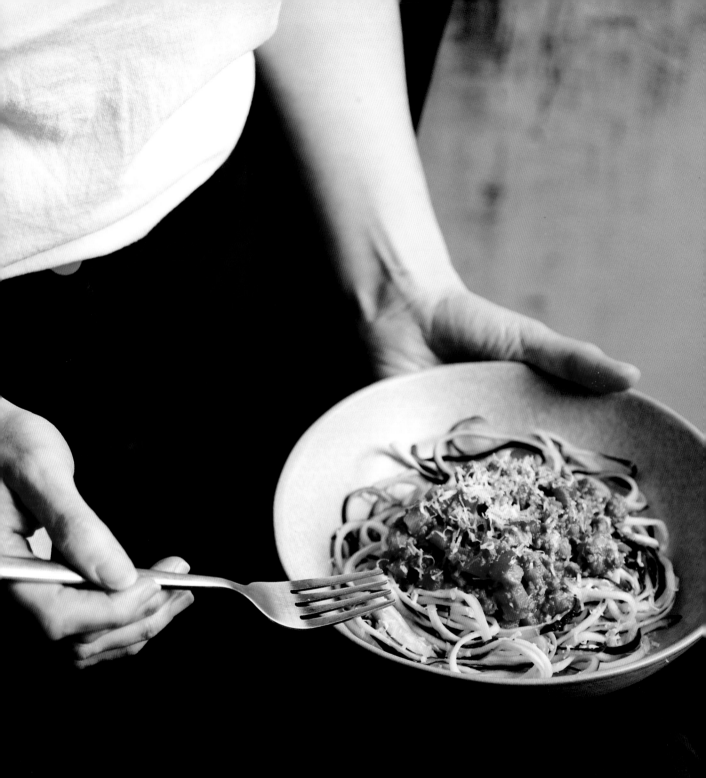

PORK PAD THAI

SERVES
1

PREPARATION
10 MINS

COOK
10 MINS

COST PER SERVE
$2.50

50 g wide rice noodles
½ teaspoon sambal oelek (chilli paste)
½ garlic clove, grated
1 teaspoon rice wine vinegar
½ teaspoon pure maple syrup
½ teaspoon fish sauce
1 teaspoon lime juice
1 teaspoon coconut oil
60 g pork fillet, finely sliced
1 free-range egg, lightly beaten
1 carrot, grated
½ cup bean sprouts, trimmed
2 teaspoons chopped unsalted cashews
1 tablespoon coriander leaves
½ spring onion, sliced

Cook the noodles according to packet directions. Drain and set aside. (Rinse in cold water to make pliable again before frying.)

Meanwhile, combine the sambal oelek, garlic, rice wine vinegar, maple syrup, fish sauce and lime juice in a bowl to make a sauce.

Heat the coconut oil in a non-stick frying pan over medium–high heat. Add the pork and cook for 2–3 minutes until cooked through. Remove from the pan and set aside.

Add the drained noodles and sauce to the pan and toss to coat. Toss through the beaten egg until cooked through.

Return the pork to the pan, add the carrot and bean sprouts and toss everything together over the heat for 1 minute.

Transfer the mixture to a bowl, top with the chopped cashews, coriander leaves and spring onion and serve.

NUTRI DETAILS PER SERVE

1272 kJ/303 cals	Sat fat: 7.1 g
Protein: 22.9 g	Carbs: 18.6 g
Fibre: 3.7 g	Total sugar: 6.7 g
Total fat: 14.3 g	Free sugar: 2 g

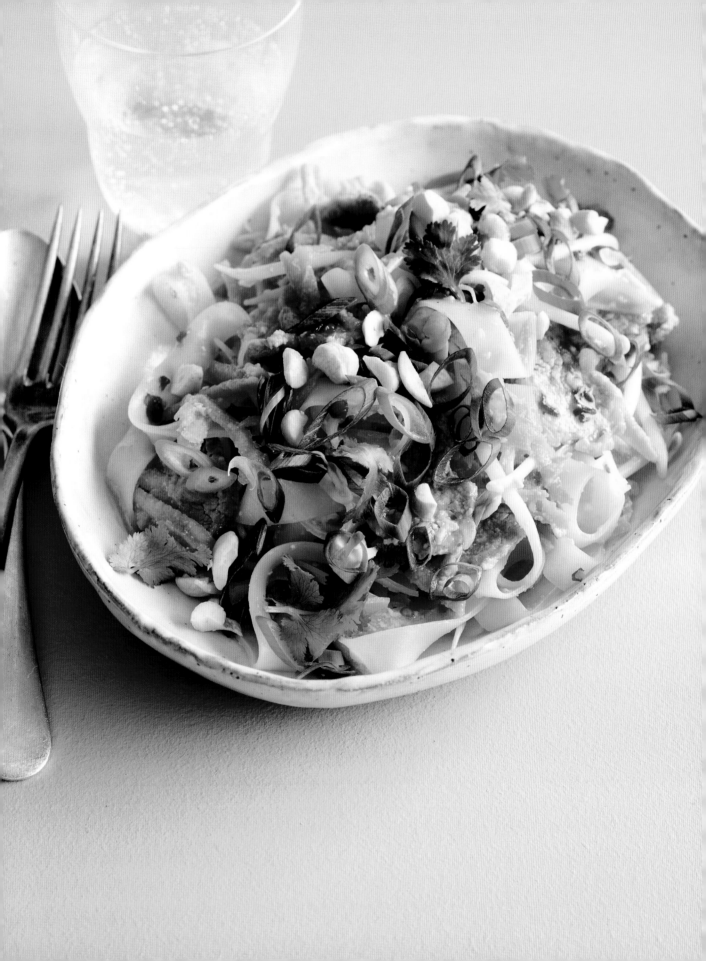

STOVETOP

Simply delicious dinners!

MEXICAN QUINOA, CHICKPEA AND CORN CASSEROLE

SERVES
4

PREPARATION
10 MINS

COOK
20 MINS

COST PER SERVE
$1.93

1 teaspoon extra-virgin olive oil

1 brown onion, diced

1 red capsicum, diced

1 cup quinoa, rinsed

1 × 400 g can chickpeas, drained and rinsed

1 × 400 g can diced tomatoes

1 cup corn kernels (fresh or canned)

2 teaspoons dried chilli flakes

2 teaspoons ground cumin

½ lime

2 tablespoons coriander leaves

1 avocado, mashed

Heat the olive oil in a flameproof casserole dish or a large, deep frying pan over medium heat. Add the onion and capsicum and cook for 3 minutes until softened.

Add the quinoa, chickpeas, tomatoes, corn, chilli flakes, cumin and 2 cups of water and stir well to combine. Increase the heat to medium–high and cook, covered, for 15 minutes until the quinoa is tender.

Transfer the quinoa mixture to a serving dish, if necessary. Finish with a squeeze of lime juice and a sprinkling of coriander and serve with the mashed avocado on the side.

Store any leftovers in an airtight container in the fridge for 3–4 days or freeze for up to 3 months.

SUITABLE TO FREEZE

NUTRI DETAILS PER SERVE

1706 kJ/408 cals	Sat fat: 1.6 g
Protein: 15.8 g	Carbs: 54 g
Fibre: 13 g	Total sugar: 8.5 g
Total fat: 10.4 g	Free sugar: 0 g

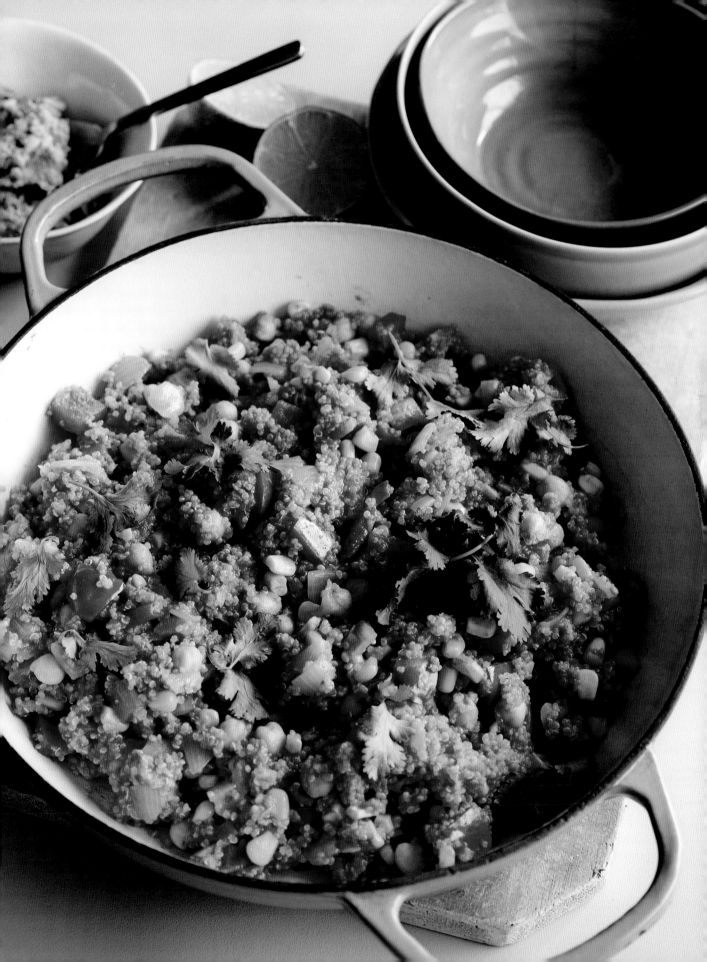

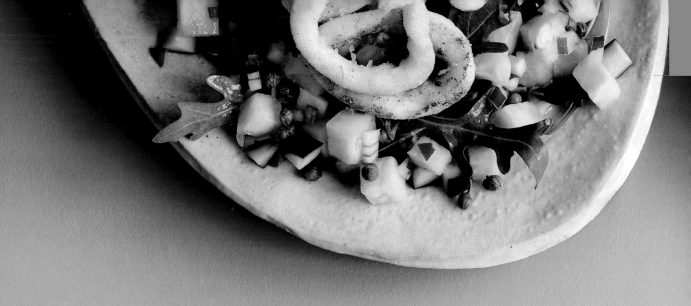

FLASH-FRIED SQUID WITH ROCKET AND PINEAPPLE

SERVES
4

PREPARATION
10 MINS

COOK
5 MINS

COST PER SERVE
$2.50

⅔ cup wholemeal plain flour
2 tablespoons finely grated
   lemon zest
freshly ground black pepper
480 g cleaned squid tubes,
   sliced into rings
2 tablespoons extra-virgin
   olive oil
60 g rocket leaves
1 Lebanese cucumber, diced
2 tablespoons baby capers,
   rinsed
½ red onion, finely diced
160 g pineapple (fresh or
   canned), diced
⅓ cup lemon juice
salt

Combine the flour and lemon zest in a bowl and season with pepper. Dust the squid rings in the flour mixture, shaking off the excess.

Heat the olive oil in a frying pan or wok over high heat. Add the squid rings and flash-fry for 1–2 minutes. Set aside.

Meanwhile, combine the rocket, cucumber, capers, red onion and pineapple in a bowl. Dress with the lemon juice and season with salt and pepper. Serve topped with the squid.

NUTRI DETAILS PER SERVE

1236 kJ/294 cals	Sat fat: 1.8 g
Protein: 32 g	Carbs: 21.7 g
Fibre: 4.4 g	Total sugar: 7.6 g
Total fat: 11.3 g	Free sugar: 0 g

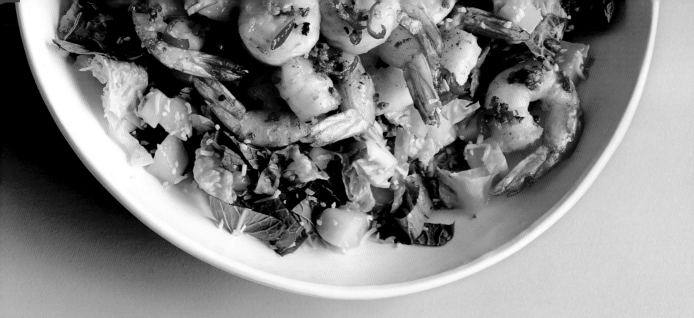

MANGO, COCONUT AND CHILLI PRAWNS

SERVES
4

PREPARATION
10 MINS

COOK
5 MINS

COST PER SERVE
$2.50

⅓ cup coconut oil

400 g raw prawns, peeled and deveined, tails intact

4 garlic cloves, crushed

3 bird's eye chillies, halved and seeds removed, finely chopped (optional)

4 cheeks mango, diced

⅓ cup shredded coconut, toasted

⅓ cup lime juice

⅓ cup chopped mint leaves

120 g cos lettuce leaves, chopped

1 tablespoon sesame seeds, toasted

Heat the coconut oil in a frying pan over medium–high heat. Add the prawns, garlic and chilli (if using) and cook for 2–3 minutes on each side until the prawns are cooked through. Set aside.

Combine the mango, coconut, lime juice, mint, lettuce and sesame seeds in a bowl. Top with the prawns and serve.

NUTRI DETAILS PER SERVE

1706 kJ/406 cals	Sat fat: 23 g
Protein: 24 g	Carbs: 15.5 g
Fibre: 5 g	Total sugar: 14 g
Total fat: 26.7 g	Free sugar: 0 g

CHICKEN AND CORN FRITTERS

SERVES
4

PREPARATION
10 MINS, PLUS
COOLING TIME

COOK
20 MINS

COST PER SERVE
$2.42

cooking oil spray
200 g chicken breast fillet
1 cup reduced-fat milk
  of choice
4 free-range eggs
1⅓ cups wholemeal plain
  flour
2 teaspoons baking powder
⅓ cup grated reduced-fat
  cheddar
1⅓ cups corn kernels
  (fresh or canned)
2 teaspoons chopped chives
120 g mixed lettuce leaves
2 tomatoes, chopped
1 Lebanese cucumber,
  chopped
1¼ tablespoons lemon juice
salt and freshly ground
  black pepper
⅔ cup reduced-fat plain
  Greek yoghurt

NUTRI DETAILS PER SERVE

2007 kJ/478 cals	Sat fat: 6.6 g
Protein: 38.5 g	Carbs: 38.8 g
Fibre: 6.7 g	Total sugar: 10.9 g
Total fat: 17 g	Free sugar: 0 g

Lightly spray a large non-stick frying pan with cooking oil and heat over medium heat. Add the chicken and cook for 4–5 minutes on each side until cooked through. Set aside to cool, then shred the meat with two forks.

Whisk the milk and eggs in a medium bowl. Add the flour and baking powder and whisk until smooth and combined, then stir in the grated cheese, corn, chives and shredded chicken.

Spray the frying pan with a little more cooking oil and heat over medium–high heat.

Add ¼ cup of batter for each fritter to the pan and cook for 2–3 minutes on each side until golden and cooked through. You should have enough batter to make two or three fritters per serve. Cook them in batches if necessary.

Meanwhile, combine the lettuce, tomato and cucumber in a bowl. Dress with the lemon juice and season with salt and pepper.

Mix the yoghurt with 2 tablespoons of water and season with salt and pepper.

Divide the fritters and salad among four plates. Dollop on the yoghurt and serve.

Store any leftover fritters in an airtight container in the fridge for 2–3 days or freeze for up to 2 months.

FRITTERS ARE SUITABLE TO FREEZE

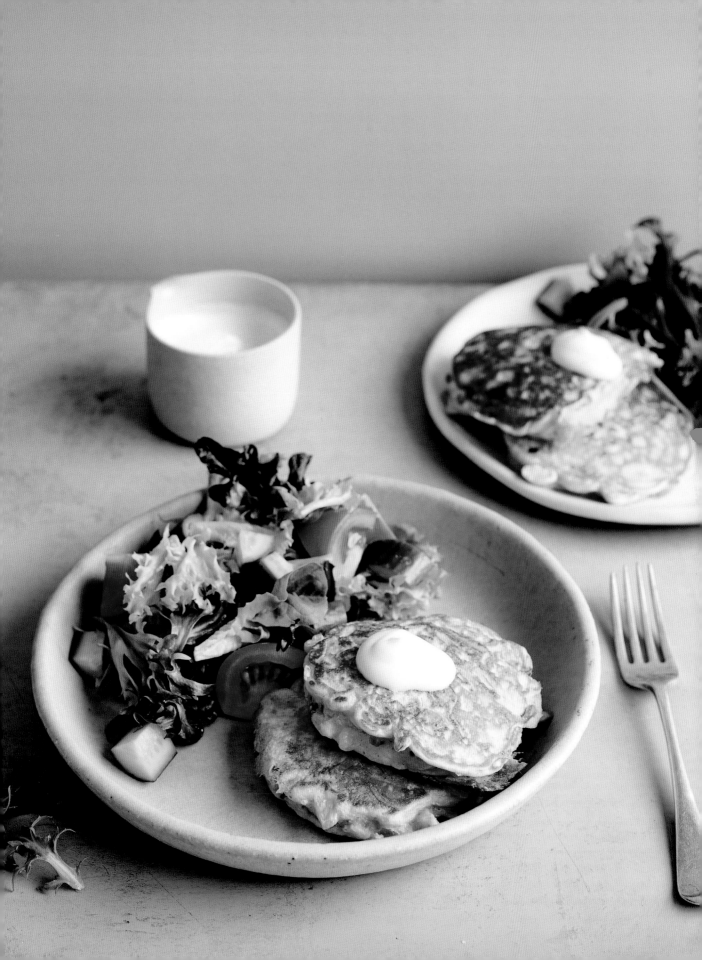

CHEESY CHICKEN MEATBALLS IN TOMATO AND SPINACH SAUCE

SERVES
4

PREPARATION
10 MINS

COOK
30 MINS

COST PER SERVE
$2.50

350 g lean chicken mince
2 carrots, grated, plus extra
if needed
½ cup grated reduced-fat
cheddar
3 free-range eggs, lightly
beaten
salt and freshly ground
black pepper
2 tablespoons extra-virgin
olive oil
1 brown onion, finely diced
800 g canned diced tomatoes
1 cup frozen peas
120 g baby spinach leaves

NUTRI DETAILS PER SERVE

1722 kJ/410 cals	Sat fat: 5.7 g
Protein: 34 g	Carbs: 13.3 g
Fibre: 6.9 g	Total sugar: 10.1 g
Total fat: 23.2 g	Free sugar: 0 g

Place the chicken mince, carrot, cheese and egg in a bowl, season with salt and pepper and mix well. Add a little more carrot if the mixture doesn't bind together well.

Heat the olive oil in a large frying pan over medium heat. Add the onion and cook for 1–2 minutes until translucent.

Add dollops of the chicken mixture to form approximately 24 meatballs. Cook for 1–2 minutes on each side to brown.

Add the canned tomatoes and bring to the boil, then reduce the heat and simmer for 15–20 minutes until the meatballs are cooked through and the sauce has thickened slightly.

Add the peas and spinach to the sauce and cook for a further 4–5 minutes until the peas are tender and the spinach has wilted.

Divide evenly among four bowls and serve.

Store any leftover meatballs and sauce in an airtight container in the fridge for 3–4 days or freeze for up to 3 months.

SUITABLE TO FREEZE

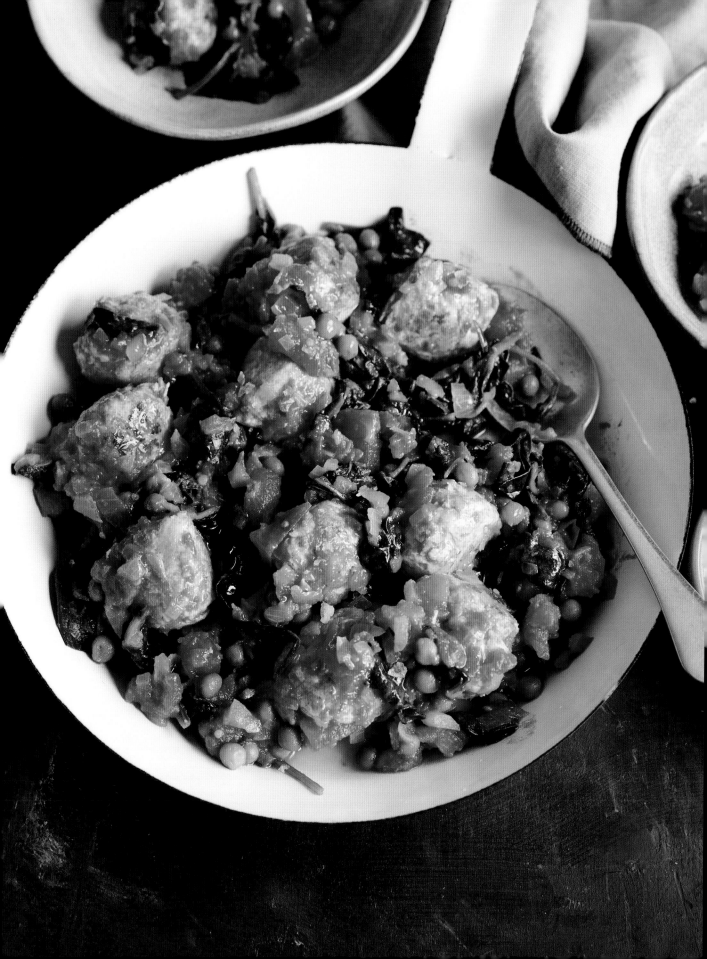

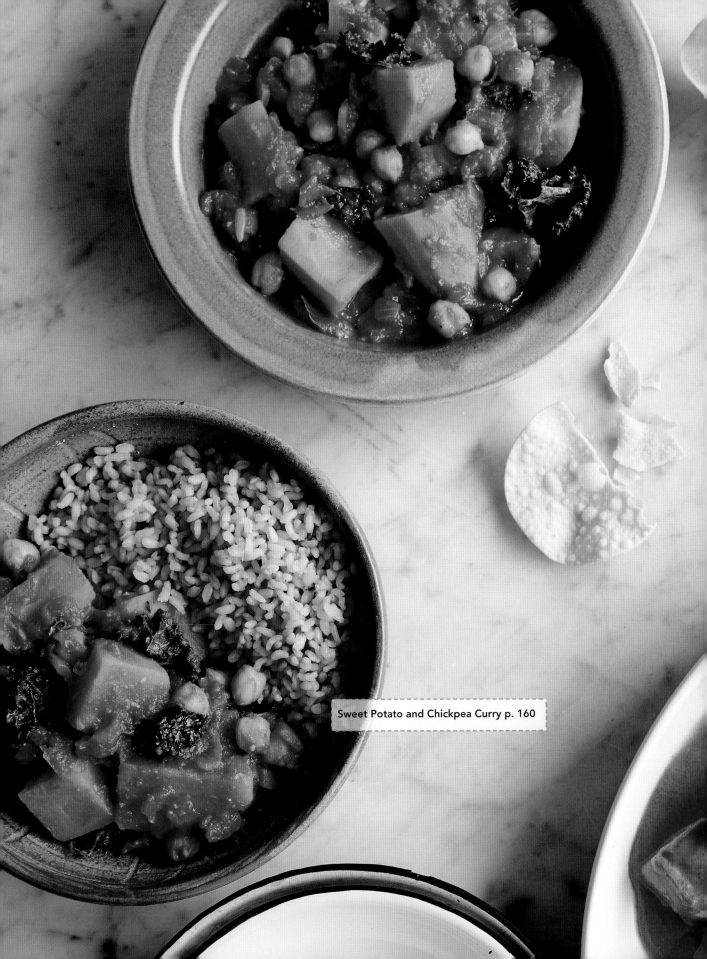

Sweet Potato and Chickpea Curry p. 160

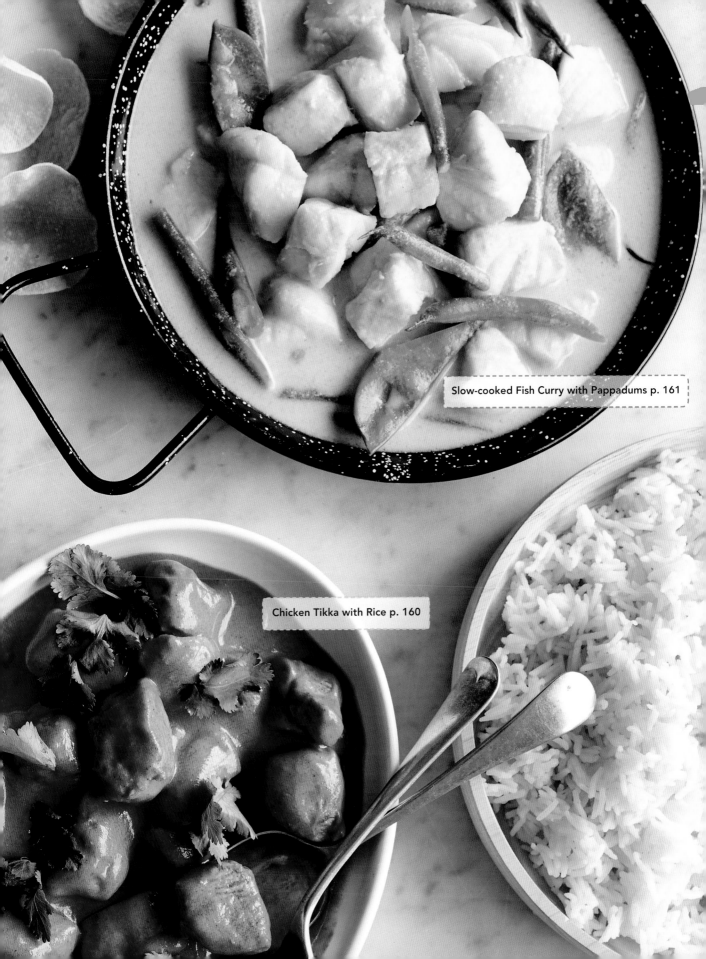

Slow-cooked Fish Curry with Pappadums p. 161

Chicken Tikka with Rice p. 160

CHICKEN TIKKA WITH RICE

SERVES
4

PREPARATION
10 MINS

COOK
15 MINS

COST PER SERVE
$1.77

1 cup basmati rice
1 tablespoon coconut oil
1 teaspoon ground cinnamon
1 teaspoon ground cumin
2 teaspoons smoked paprika
400 g chicken breast fillets, cut into bite-sized cubes
½ cup tomato paste
1⅓ cups reduced-fat coconut milk
⅓ cup coriander leaves

Bring 1 litre of water to the boil in a medium saucepan, add the rice and simmer for 10–12 minutes until tender. Drain. You could use pre-cooked rice for this recipe if you have some on hand. Just warm it through first.

Meanwhile, heat the coconut oil in a heavy-based saucepan over medium heat. Add the cinnamon, cumin and paprika and stir for 30 seconds until fragrant.

Add the chicken and brown for 1 minute. Add the tomato paste and coconut milk, then reduce the heat to low and simmer for 5–7 minutes until the sauce has thickened and the chicken is cooked through.

Divide the rice evenly among four bowls and top with the chicken and sauce. Sprinkle with the coriander and serve.

Store any leftover chicken tikka and rice in an airtight container in the fridge for 2–3 days or freeze for up to 3 months.

SUITABLE TO FREEZE

NUTRI DETAILS PER SERVE

1935 kJ/460 cals
Protein: 25.7 g
Fibre: 2.7 g
Total fat: 20.4 g

Sat fat: 12.7 g
Carbs: 42.4 g
Total sugar: 6.8 g
Free sugar: 0 g

SWEET POTATO AND CHICKPEA CURRY

SERVES
4

PREPARATION
10 MINS

COOK
25 MINS

COST PER SERVE
$1.18

⅔ cup brown rice
1 tablespoon extra-virgin olive oil
1 brown onion, diced
4 garlic cloves, crushed
1 tablespoon curry powder
200 ml salt-reduced vegetable stock
600 g canned diced tomatoes
1 × 400 g can chickpeas, drained and rinsed
2 small sweet potatoes, peeled and cubed
120 g kale leaves, shredded

Bring 3 cups of water to the boil in a medium saucepan, add the rice and simmer for 25 minutes until tender. Drain. You could use pre-cooked rice for this recipe if you have some on hand. Just warm it through first.

Meanwhile, heat the olive oil in a frying pan over medium–high heat, add the onion and cook for 2–3 minutes until softened. Add the garlic and curry powder and cook for 1 minute, then add the stock and canned tomatoes and bring to the boil.

Stir in the chickpeas and sweet potato. Reduce the heat and simmer, covered, for 10–15 minutes until the sweet potato is tender. Add the kale leaves in the final 5 minutes of cooking and allow to wilt.

Divide the rice and curry evenly among four bowls and serve.

Store any leftover rice and curry in an airtight container in the fridge for 2–3 days or freeze for up to 3 months.

SUITABLE TO FREEZE

NUTRI DETAILS PER SERVE

1591 kJ/379 cals
Protein: 17.1 g
Fibre: 15.7 g
Total fat: 3.4 g

Sat fat: 0.4 g
Carbs: 62.7 g
Total sugar: 16.2 g
Free sugar: 0 g

SLOW-COOKED FISH CURRY
WITH PAPPADUMS

SERVES
4

PREPARATION
10 MINS

COOK
20 MINS (2 HOURS 30 MINS
IN A SLOW COOKER)

COST PER SERVE
$2.50

1 tablespoon yellow
   curry paste
1 × 400 ml can reduced-fat
   coconut milk
600 g white fish fillet of
   choice, skinless and
   boneless, cut into
   bite-sized cubes
240 g green beans, trimmed
240 g snow peas, trimmed
12 mini pappadums

NUTRI DETAILS PER SERVE

1279 kJ/304 cals	Sat fat: 5.4 g
Protein: 36.5 g	Carbs: 10.3 g
Fibre: 4.7 g	Total sugar: 2.5 g
Total fat: 11.5 g	Free sugar: 0 g

If cooking on the stovetop:

Heat a heavy-based saucepan or flameproof casserole dish over medium–high heat, add the curry paste and cook for a few seconds until fragrant. Add the coconut milk and stir to combine. Add the fish, bring to the boil, then reduce the heat and simmer for 15 minutes until the fish is cooked through. Add the beans and snow peas in the final 5 minutes of cooking and cook until the veggies are tender crisp.

If cooking in a slow cooker:

Place the curry paste and coconut milk in the slow cooker dish and stir to combine. Add the fish and cook on low for 2 hours. Add the beans and snow peas and cook for a further 30 minutes.

To serve:

Divide the curry evenly among four bowls. Serve with three mini pappadums per person.

Store any leftover curry in an airtight container in the fridge for 3–4 days or freeze for up to 2 months.

SUITABLE TO FREEZE

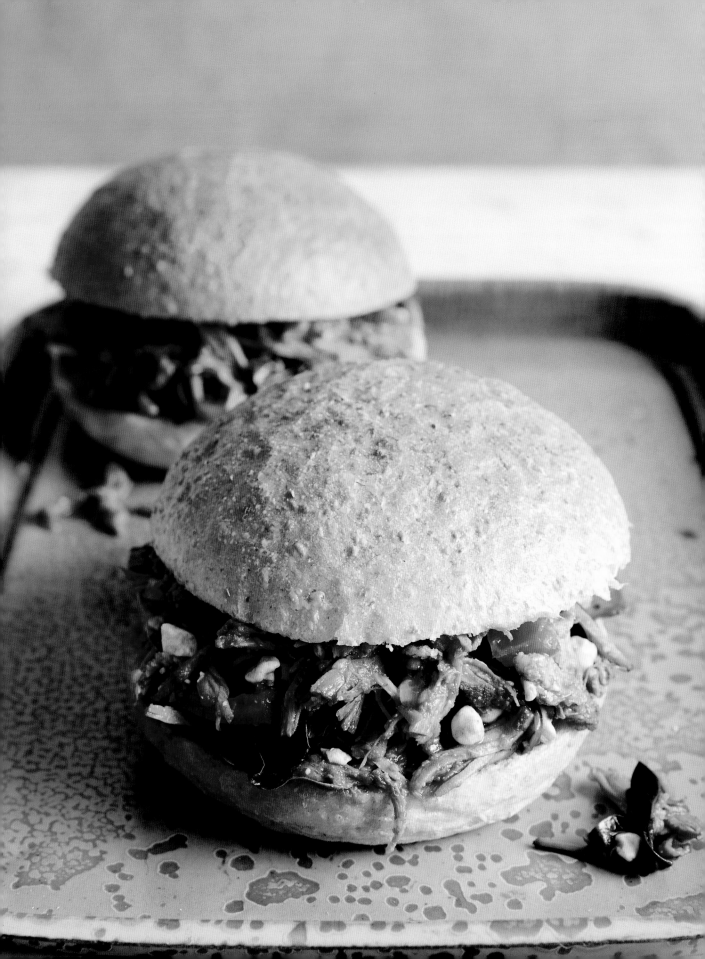

PULLED PORK AND SPINACH SLOPPY JOES

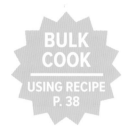

BULK COOK

USING RECIPE
P. 38

SERVES
5

PREPARATION
5 MINS

COOK
5 MINS, PLUS
BASE RECIPE

COST PER SERVE
$1.44

---

1 x quantity **Pulled Pork**
(see p. 38)
1½ tablespoons **reduced-fat
cottage cheese**
45 g **baby spinach leaves**
1½ **tomatoes, diced**
5 **wholemeal rolls**

NUTRI DETAILS PER SERVE

1453 kJ/346 cals	Sat fat: 3.8 g
Protein: 31 g	Carbs: 27.9 g
Fibre: 3.7 g	Total sugar: 6 g
Total fat: 11.6 g	Free sugar: 3.3 g

Reheat the pulled pork in the microwave or on the stovetop until warmed through.

Add the cottage cheese, baby spinach and tomato to the warmed pork and stir until well combined and the spinach has wilted.

Slice open the rolls and fill with an even amount of the pork and spinach mixture. Serve one pork roll per person.

Store any leftover pulled pork in an airtight container in the fridge for 3–4 days or freeze for up to 3 months.

OPEN BURGER WITH THE LOT

SERVES
4

PREPARATION
10 MINS

COOK
15 MINS

COST PER SERVE
$2.30

---

480 g lean beef mince
salt and freshly ground
    black pepper
1 tablespoon extra-virgin
    olive oil
4 slices reduced-fat cheddar
4 free-range eggs
4 slices wholegrain
    sourdough bread
60 g baby spinach leaves
1 tomato, sliced
8 slices canned beetroot,
    drained
⅓ cup sauerkraut
1 teaspoon dried chilli flakes
    (optional)

NUTRI DETAILS PER SERVE

1786 kJ/425 cals	Sat fat: 6.3 g
Protein: 43 g	Carbs: 21.7 g
Fibre: 3.8 g	Total sugar: 4.7 g
Total fat: 17 g	Free sugar: 0 g

Season the beef mince with salt and pepper and shape into four even-sized patties.

Heat the olive oil in a frying pan over medium–high heat. Add the patties and cook for 4–5 minutes on each side until cooked through.

About 1 minute before the patties are ready, top each one with a slice of cheese and allow the cheese to melt. Remove from the pan and set aside to rest.

Crack the eggs into the hot frying pan and cook for 1–2 minutes or until cooked to your liking.

Toast the sourdough and top each slice with some baby spinach, tomato and beetroot. Add a burger patty and fried egg and top with a good spoonful of sauerkraut and a sprinkling of chilli flakes (if using). Serve.

Store any leftover cooked or uncooked burger patties in an airtight container in the fridge for 2–3 days or freeze for up to 3 months.

BURGER PATTIES ARE SUITABLE TO FREEZE

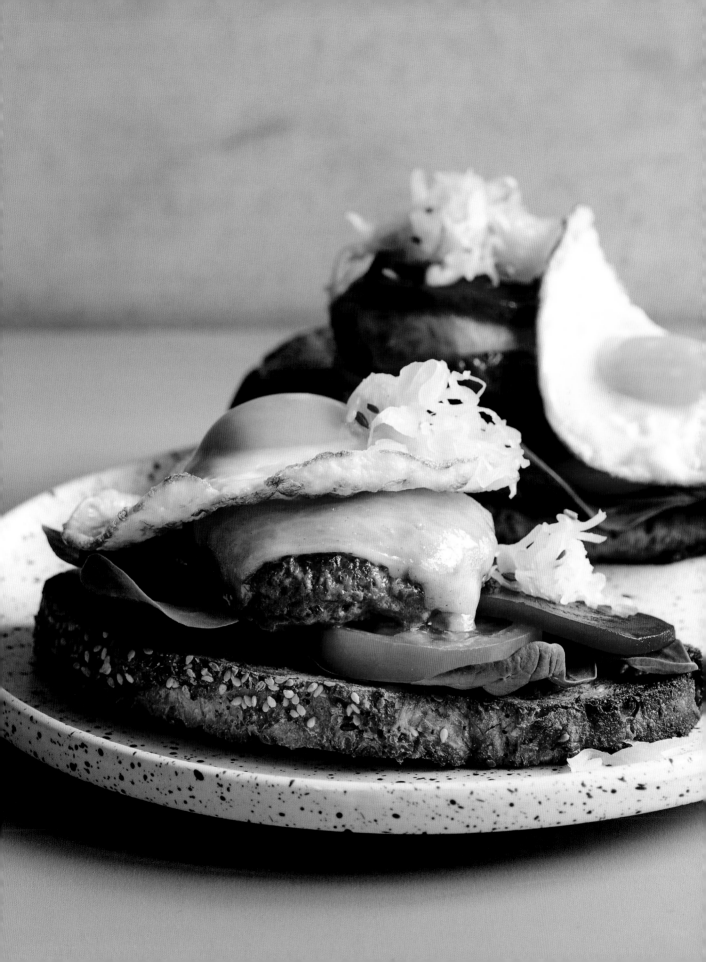

BEEF CHOW MEIN

SERVES
4

PREPARATION
10 MINS

COOK
20 MINS

COST PER SERVE
$1.53

1 tablespoon coconut oil
400 g lean beef mince
salt and freshly ground
   black pepper
1 cup salt-reduced
   chicken stock
2 carrots, grated
200 g white cabbage, chopped
240 g green beans, trimmed
   and halved
2 tablespoons tamari
   (gluten-free soy sauce)

Heat the coconut oil in a frying pan over medium–high heat. Add the mince and cook, breaking up any lumps with the back of a wooden spoon, for 4–5 minutes until the meat is browned all over. Season with salt and pepper.

Add the chicken stock, carrot, cabbage and beans and bring to the boil, then reduce the heat and simmer for 10 minutes until the veggies are tender and most of the liquid has been absorbed.

Add the tamari and simmer for a further 1–2 minutes, then divide among four bowls and serve.

NUTRI DETAILS PER SERVE

935 kJ/223 cals	Sat fat: 4.5 g
Protein: 26 g	Carbs: 5.9 g
Fibre: 5 g	Total sugar: 4.8 g
Total fat: 9.4 g	Free sugar: 0 g

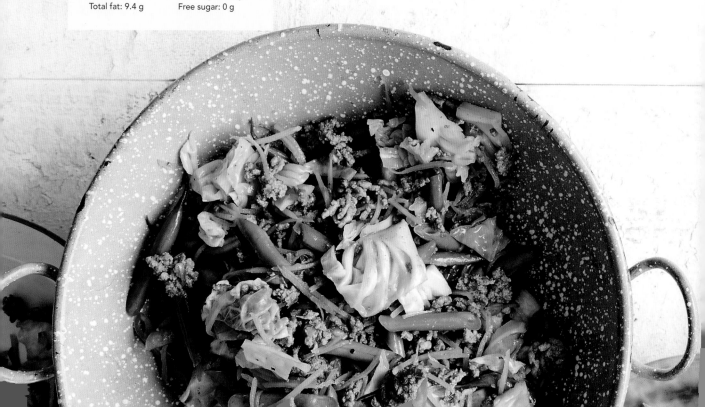

CHICKEN BURRITO BOWLS

SERVES
4

PREPARATION
10 MINS

COOK
25 MINS

COST PER SERVE
$2.44

1 cup brown rice
1 tablespoon extra-virgin olive oil
320 g chicken breast fillet, sliced
1 teaspoon cayenne pepper
1 tablespoon lemon juice
75 g mushrooms, sliced
1 cup corn kernels (fresh or canned)
1 × 400 g can black beans, drained and rinsed
4 tomatoes, diced
1 green capsicum, sliced
⅓ cup coriander leaves

Bring 1 litre of water to the boil in a medium saucepan, add the rice and simmer for 25 minutes until tender. Drain. You could use pre-cooked rice for this recipe if you have some on hand. Just warm it through first.

Meanwhile, heat the olive oil in a frying pan over medium–high heat. Season the chicken with the cayenne pepper and add to the pan along with the lemon juice. Cook for 5–7 minutes until the chicken is cooked through. Add the mushroom during the final 2 minutes of cooking and cook until tender.

When the rice is ready, place an even amount in one section of four serving bowls. Place an even amount of chicken and mushroom in another section, followed by even portions of corn, black beans, tomato and capsicum. Sprinkle the coriander over the top and serve.

NUTRI DETAILS PER SERVE

1729 kJ/395 cals	Sat fat: 1.5 g
Protein: 30.2 g	Carbs: 48 g
Fibre: 11 g	Total sugar: 8.7 g
Total fat: 8.7 g	Free sugar: 0 g

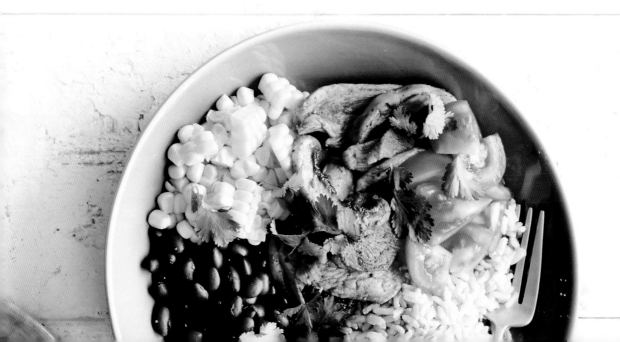

BEEF STROGANOFF WITH POLENTA

SERVES
4

PREPARATION
10 MINS

COOK
45 MINS

COST PER SERVE
$2.46

½ cup fine polenta
cooking oil spray
360 g lean beef rump,
    finely sliced
1 brown onion, sliced
150 g mushrooms, sliced
1 tablespoon plain
    wholemeal flour
1 cup salt-reduced beef stock
1 tablespoon tomato paste
1 tablespoon Worcestershire
    sauce
½ cup reduced-fat plain
    Greek yoghurt
120 g green beans, trimmed

NUTRI DETAILS PER SERVE

1104 kJ/263 cals
Protein: 26.7 g
Fibre: 3.3 g
Total fat: 5.6 g

Sat fat: 2.3 g
Carbs: 24.3 g
Total sugar: 5.7 g
Free sugar: 0.4 g

Pour 1 litre of water into a saucepan and bring to the boil over medium–high heat. While gently whisking the water, pour the polenta into the boiling water in a steady stream. Continue whisking for 5–7 minutes until the polenta has thickened (check the packet directions to be on the safe side).

Reduce the heat to low and continue whisking until the polenta has thickened enough so that it doesn't settle back on the base of the pan when you stop stirring. Cover and cook over very low heat for 25 minutes, stirring vigorously every 5 minutes or so, making sure you scrape the side and base of the pan.

Meanwhile, lightly spray a frying pan with cooking oil and heat over medium heat. Add the beef and cook for 3–4 minutes for medium–rare or until cooked to your liking. Remove the beef and set aside.

Reduce the heat to medium–low, add the onion and mushroom to the pan and cook for about 5 minutes or until the mushroom is tender. Stir in the flour and cook for a further minute, then add the stock, tomato paste and Worcestershire sauce and stir to combine.

Return the beef to the pan and simmer for 5 minutes until the sauce has thickened and reduced slightly. Remove from the heat and stir through the yoghurt.

Steam the beans in the microwave or on the stovetop for 2–3 minutes or until tender.

Divide the stroganoff among four plates and serve with an even portion of polenta and beans on the side. Store any leftovers in an airtight container in the fridge for 2–3 days or freeze the beef and polenta for up to 3 months.

BEEF AND POLENTA SUITABLE TO FREEZE

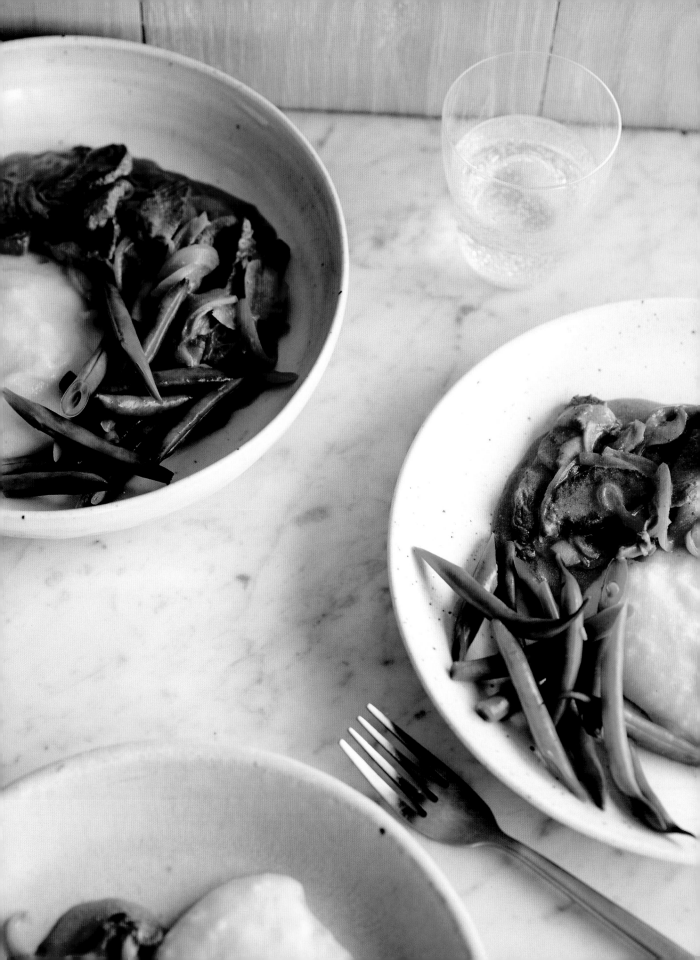

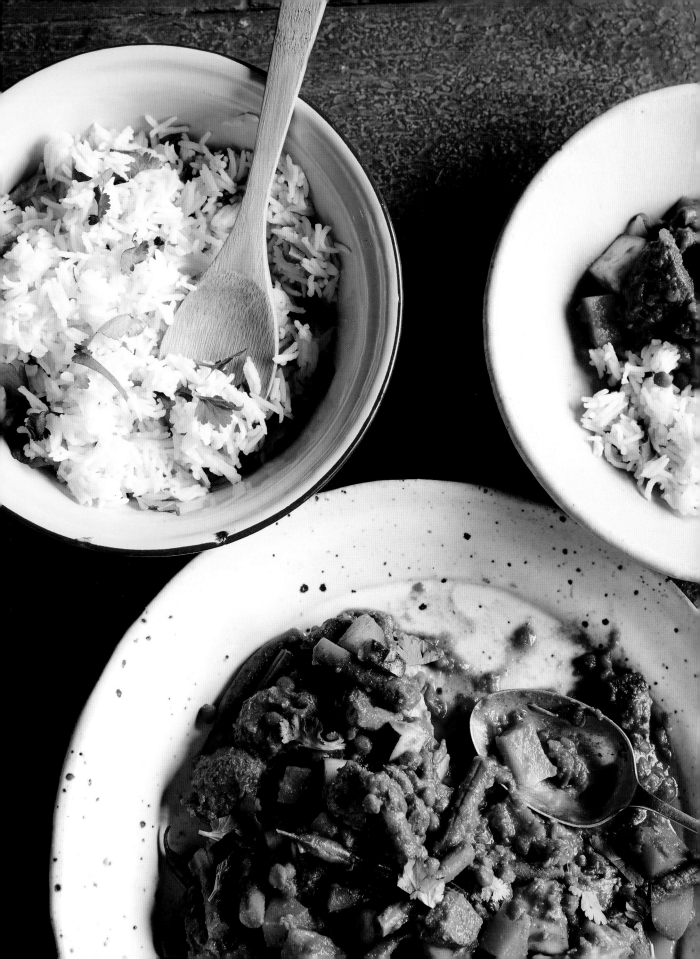

LAMB AND LENTIL CURRY WITH CORIANDER RICE

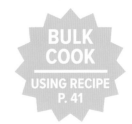

BULK COOK
USING RECIPE P. 41

SERVES
4

PREPARATION
5 MINS

COOK
15 MINS, PLUS BASE RECIPE

COST PER SERVE
$2.32

¾ cup basmati rice
2 tablespoons chopped coriander leaves
1 x quantity Lamb and Lentil Curry (see p. 41)
2 tablespoons reduced-fat plain Greek yoghurt

NUTRI DETAILS PER SERVE

1861kJ/443 cals	Sat fat: 3.3 g
Protein: 29.2 g	Carbs: 51 g
Fibre: 8.4 g	Total sugar: 7.0 g
Total fat: 11.4 g	Free sugar: 0 g

FOR A VEGETARIAN MEAL

Omit the lamb, use vegetable stock and add 320 g cubed sweet potato and a drained 400 g can of corn kernels to the curry.

COST PER SERVE $1.91

Bring 3 cups of water to the boil in a medium saucepan, add the rice and simmer for 10–12 minutes until tender. Drain and stir in most of the coriander, saving some to garnish.

Meanwhile, reheat the lamb and lentil curry in the microwave or on the stovetop until warmed through.

Divide the curry and coriander rice evenly among four bowls, top with a dollop of yoghurt, sprinkle with the remaining coriander and serve.

Store any leftover curry in an airtight container in the fridge for 4–5 days or freeze for up to 3 months.

BAKES

Straight from the oven to the table!

LENTIL SHEPHERD'S PIE

SERVES
4

PREPARATION
10 MINS

COOK
35 MINS

COST PER SERVE
$1.75

---

2 × 400 g cans brown lentils,
    drained and rinsed
2 cups tomato passata
2 carrots, diced
1 cup frozen peas
salt and freshly ground
    black pepper
2 small sweet potatoes,
    peeled and diced
⅔ cup grated reduced-fat
    cheddar

NUTRI DETAILS PER SERVE

1534 kJ/365 cals	Sat fat: 1.4 g
Protein: 27 g	Carbs: 47.5 g
Fibre: 17 g	Total sugar: 18.5 g
Total fat: 3.4 g	Free sugar: 0 g

Preheat the oven to 190°C.

Combine the lentils, passata, carrot and peas in a saucepan over medium heat and season with salt and pepper. Bring to the boil, then reduce the heat and simmer for 20 minutes, adding a little water if the mixture thickens too much.

Meanwhile, cook the sweet potato in a saucepan of boiling water for 10 minutes until tender. Drain and mash.

Transfer the lentil mixture to a medium baking dish and top with the sweet potato mash. Sprinkle over the grated cheese and bake for 15 minutes until the cheese is melted and golden.

Divide evenly among four plates and serve.

Store any leftovers in an airtight container in the fridge for 3–4 days or freeze for up to 3 months.

SUITABLE TO FREEZE

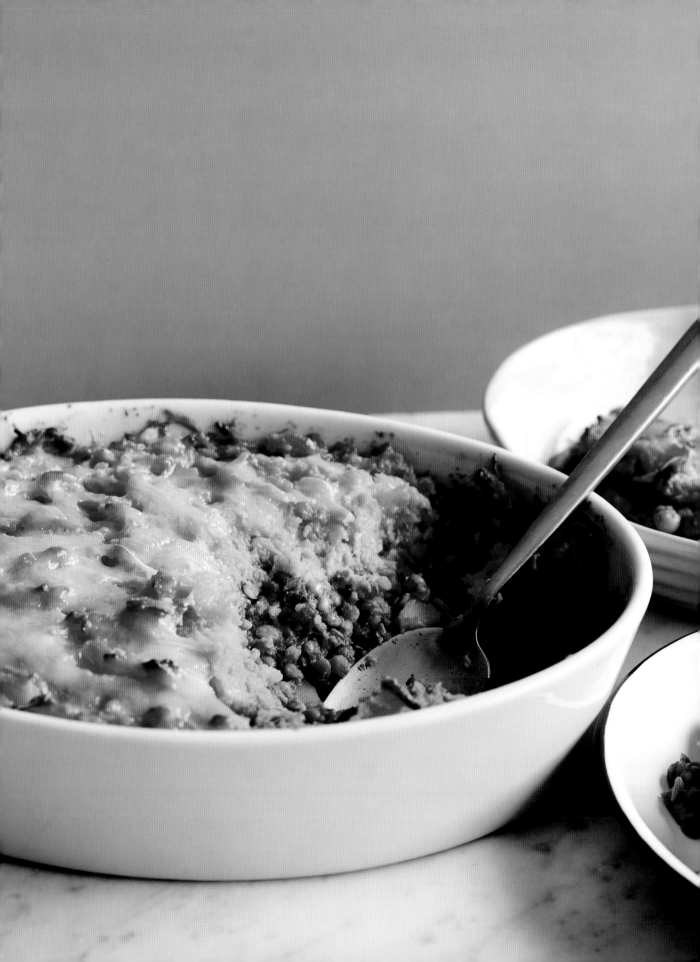

BAKED SWEET POTATOES WITH SPINACH AND FETA

SERVES
4

PREPARATION
10 MINS

COOK
45 MINS

COST PER SERVE
$2.50

4 small sweet potatoes
2 tablespoons extra-virgin
   olive oil
1 brown onion, finely sliced
240 g baby spinach leaves,
   chopped
1 teaspoon cayenne pepper
80 g reduced-fat feta
juice of ½ lemon

NUTRI DETAILS PER SERVE

1285 kJ/306 cals	Sat fat: 5 g
Protein: 15.2 g	Carbs: 24.8 g
Fibre: 4.9 g	Total sugar: 10.7 g
Total fat: 15.3 g	Free sugar: 0 g

Preheat the oven to 200°C.

Prick the sweet potatoes all over with a fork, then place in the oven and bake for 45 minutes or until tender.

When the sweet potatoes are nearly ready, heat the olive oil in a frying pan over medium–high heat. Add the onion and cook for 1–2 minutes until translucent. Add the spinach and cook for 2–3 minutes until wilted. Season with the cayenne pepper.

To serve, split each sweet potato down the centre and gently mash the flesh with a fork.

Top the sweet potatoes with an even amount of the spinach mixture, then crumble over the feta and finish with a squeeze of lemon juice. Serve.

Wrap any leftovers in foil and store in an airtight container in the fridge for 3–4 days or freeze for up to 3 months.

SUITABLE TO FREEZE

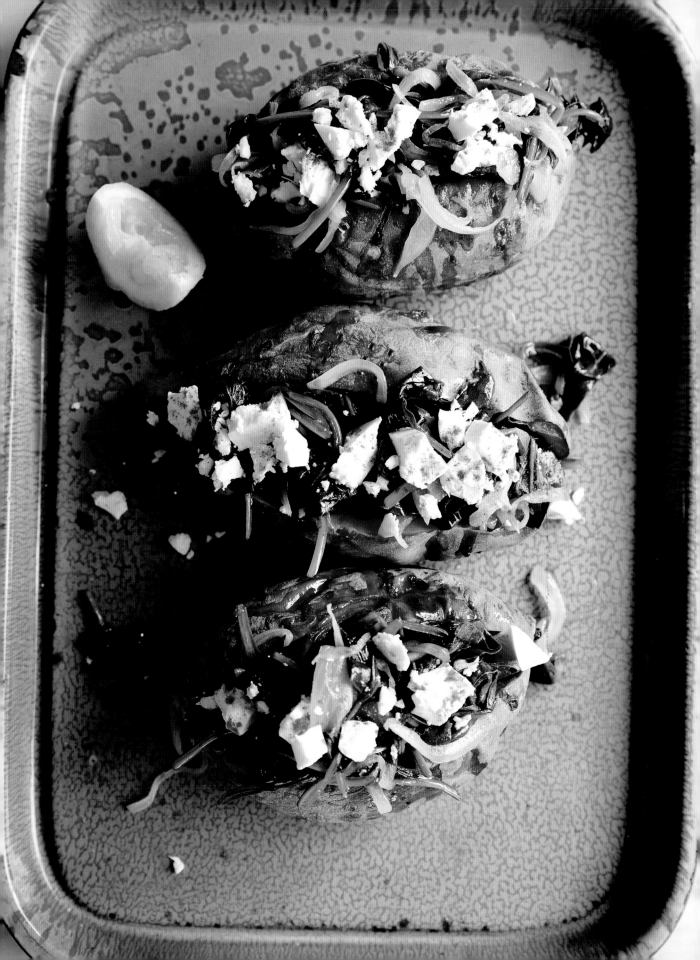

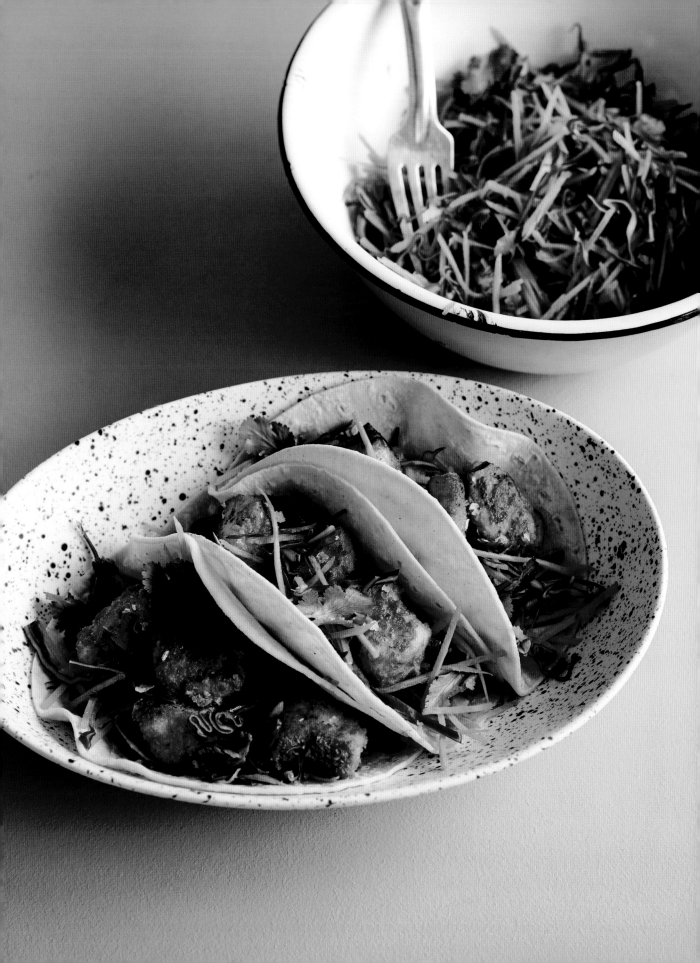

FISH TACOS WITH COLESLAW

SERVES
4

PREPARATION
10 MINS

COOK
10 MINS

COST PER SERVE
$1.86

½ cup fresh wholemeal breadcrumbs
1 teaspoon chilli powder
2 teaspoons smoked paprika
2 teaspoons ground cumin
1 teaspoon garlic powder
2 teaspoons ground turmeric
480 g white fish fillet of choice, skinless and boneless, cut into bite-sized cubes
100 g red cabbage, shredded
⅓ cup roughly chopped coriander leaves
4 carrots, grated
⅓ cup lime juice
1 tablespoon apple cider vinegar
salt and freshly ground black pepper
8 small corn tortillas

NUTRI DETAILS PER SERVE

1670 kJ/396 cals	Sat fat: 1.3 g
Protein: 30 g	Carbs: 48 g
Fibre: 6.9 g	Total sugar: 6 g
Total fat: 7.7 g	Free sugar: 0 g

Preheat the oven to 180°C and line a baking tray with baking paper.

Combine the breadcrumbs and ground spices in a bowl. Coat the fish pieces in the crumb mixture and arrange on the prepared tray. Bake for 10 minutes until the fish is cooked through, turning halfway through the cooking time.

Meanwhile, combine the cabbage, coriander, carrot, lime juice and apple cider vinegar in a bowl. Season with salt and pepper and set aside.

Warm the tortillas in the microwave for a few seconds. Assemble the tacos by topping each tortilla with some slaw and crumbed fish. Wrap to enclose the filling and serve. Two tortillas is one serve.

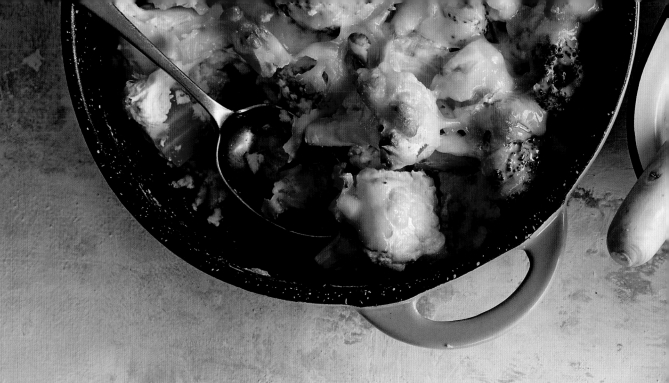

CHEESY VEGGIE BAKE

SERVES
4

PREPARATION
10 MINS

COOK
30 MINS

COST PER SERVE
$1.03

200 g broccoli, cut into
  florets
200 g cauliflower, cut into
  florets
2 carrots, diced
2 cups reduced-fat natural
  Greek-style yoghurt
2 free-range egg yolks
½ teaspoon mustard powder
1 cup grated reduced-fat
  cheddar

Preheat the oven to 180°C.

Place the broccoli, cauliflower and carrot in a baking dish.

Combine the yoghurt, egg yolks, mustard powder and half the cheese in a bowl, then fold through the vegetables.

Sprinkle with the remaining cheese and bake for 30 minutes or until golden and the vegetables are cooked through.

Divide evenly among four plates and serve.

Store any leftovers in an airtight container in the fridge for 3–4 days or freeze for up to 2 months.

SUITABLE TO FREEZE

NUTRI DETAILS PER SERVE

1739 kJ/414 cals	Sat fat: 15.5 g
Protein: 27.7 g	Carbs: 13.5 g
Fibre: 4 g	Total sugar: 13.2 g
Total fat: 26.4 g	Free sugar: 0 g

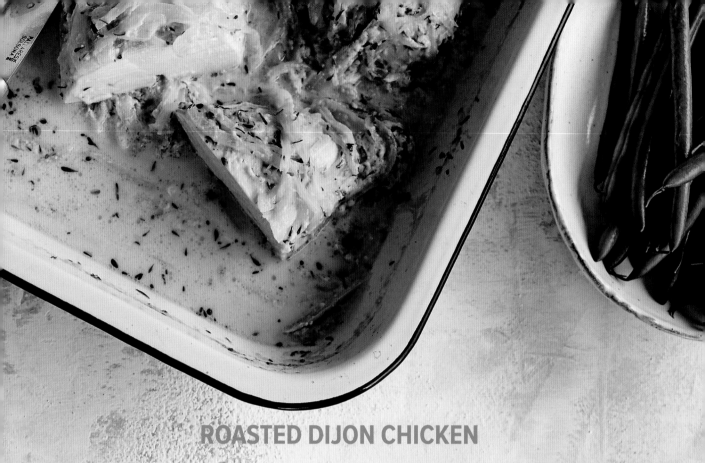

ROASTED DIJON CHICKEN

SERVES
4

PREPARATION
10 MINS

COOK
30 MINS

COST PER SERVE
$2.50

480 g chicken breast fillets
salt and freshly ground
black pepper
1 tablespoon extra-virgin
olive oil
1 brown onion, finely sliced
700 ml salt-reduced
chicken stock
200 ml reduced-fat cream
2 teaspoons dried thyme
2 tablespoons Dijon mustard
240 g green beans, trimmed

NUTRI DETAILS PER SERVE

1580 kJ/376 cals	Sat fat: 10.1 g
Protein: 32.6 g	Carbs: 8.3 g
Fibre: 3.9 g	Total sugar: 5.2 g
Total fat: 23 g	Free sugar: 0 g

Preheat the oven to 180°C.

Season the chicken with salt and pepper, place in a roasting tin and set aside.

Heat the olive oil in a frying pan over medium–high heat, add the onion and cook for 2–3 minutes until translucent. Add the stock, scraping up any brown bits from the bottom of the pan, and simmer for 5 minutes until the liquid has reduced by half. Stir in the cream and thyme. Whisk in the mustard, then pour the sauce over the chicken.

Bake for 15–20 minutes until the chicken is cooked through.

Just before the chicken is ready, steam the beans in the microwave or on the stovetop until tender crisp.

Slice the chicken into four equal-sized portions. Divide the chicken and beans evenly among four plates and serve with the Dijon sauce spooned over the top.

CHICKEN AND JALAPENO POPPERS WITH GUACAMOLE

SERVES
4

PREPARATION
15 MINS

COOK
1 HOUR (8 HOURS 10 MINS IN A SLOW COOKER)

COST PER SERVE
$2.03

---

300 g chicken breast fillet
salt and freshly ground
    black pepper
cooking oil spray
50 g light cream cheese
¼ cup sliced pickled
    jalapeno chilli
1 teaspoon garlic powder
1 teaspoon ground cumin
8 mini tortillas
½ cup grated reduced-fat
    cheddar
½ avocado, mashed
¼ cup extra-light sour cream
2 tablespoons chopped
    coriander leaves
2 tablespoons lime juice

NUTRI DETAILS PER SERVE

1389 kJ/331 cals	Sat fat: 6.2 g
Protein: 16.5 g	Carbs: 21.8 g
Fibre: 1.8 g	Total sugar: 3.2 g
Total fat: 14.9 g	Free sugar: 0 g

If cooking in the oven:
Preheat the oven to 180°C.

Season the chicken with salt and pepper and lightly spray with cooking oil. Place in a small baking dish and bake for 30–35 minutes or until cooked through. Transfer the chicken to a plate and shred with two forks.

Combine the shredded chicken, cream cheese, jalapeno, garlic powder and cumin in a bowl. Scoop the mixture into the baking dish, spread it out evenly and bake for 15 minutes.

If cooking in a slow cooker:
Lightly spray the slow cooker dish with cooking oil. Add the chicken, cream cheese, jalapeno, garlic powder, cumin and ½ cup of water and season with salt and pepper. Cover and cook on low for 6–8 hours.

Remove the chicken and shred with two forks. Return the chicken to the sauce and stir through.

To serve:
Preheat an overhead grill to high and line a baking tray with baking paper.

Heat the tortillas in the microwave for a few seconds to soften them up and make them easier to work with. Sprinkle an even amount of cheese along the middle of each tortilla and top with 2–3 tablespoons of the chicken mixture. Tightly roll up the tortillas and place on the prepared tray, seam-side down.

Grill for 8–10 minutes, turning halfway through, until the tortillas are golden and the cheese has melted.

Meanwhile, combine the avocado, sour cream, coriander and lime juice in a bowl.

Serve two poppers per person with guacamole for dipping.

Store any leftover poppers and dip in an airtight container in the fridge for 2–3 days or freeze leftover poppers for up to 2 months.

POPPERS ARE SUITABLE TO FREEZE

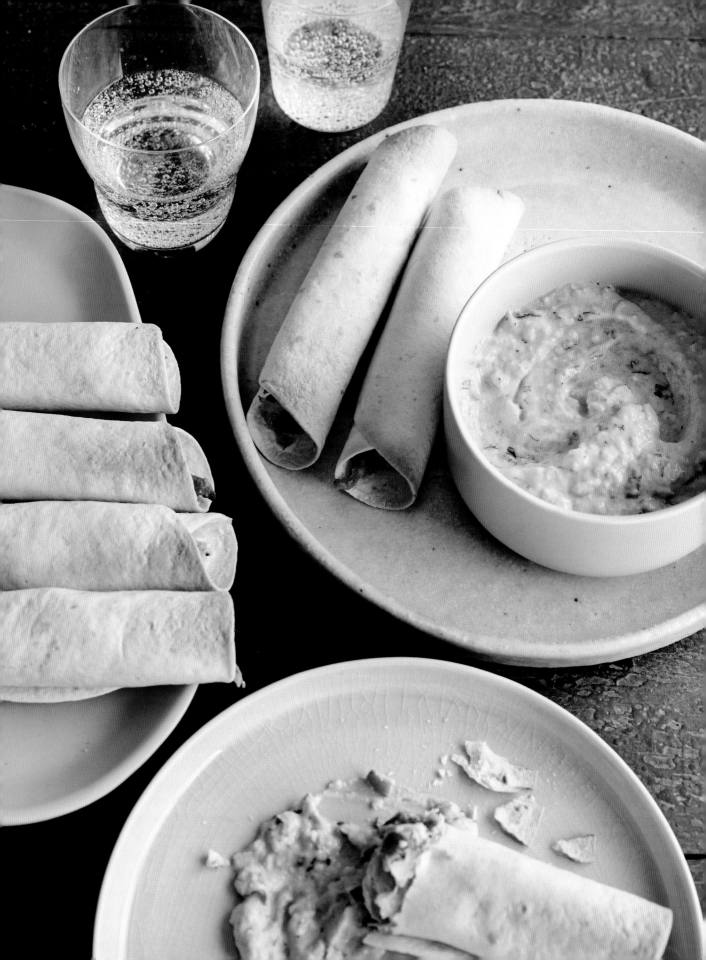

THAI CHICKEN MEATLOAF

SERVES
4

PREPARATION
10 MINS, PLUS
STANDING TIME

COOK
45 MINS

COST PER SERVE
$2.41

cooking oil spray
80 g rice vermicelli noodles
boiling water
400 g lean chicken mince
1 cup chopped coriander
   leaves
2 carrots, grated
⅓ cup sweet chilli sauce
4 free-range eggs

NUTRI DETAILS PER SERVE

1102 kJ/262 cals	Sat fat: 3.9 g
Protein: 26.8 g	Carbs: 22.8 g
Fibre: 1.8 g	Total sugar: 15.8 g
Total fat: 13.3 g	Free sugar: 13.8 g

Preheat the oven to 180°C. Lightly spray a standard loaf tin with cooking oil.

Place the vermicelli noodles in a heatproof bowl and cover with boiling water. Allow to soak for 10 minutes until the noodles are tender. Drain well, then cut into shorter lengths.

Place the noodles, chicken mince, coriander, carrot, chilli sauce and egg in a bowl. Mix with clean hands until well combined.

Transfer the mixture to the prepared tin and smooth the surface. Bake for 45 minutes until cooked through.

Slice into eight even-sized pieces and serve with a side salad, if you like. Two slices is one serve.

Store any leftover meatloaf in an airtight container in the fridge for 2–3 days or freeze in portions for up to 3 months.

SUITABLE TO FREEZE

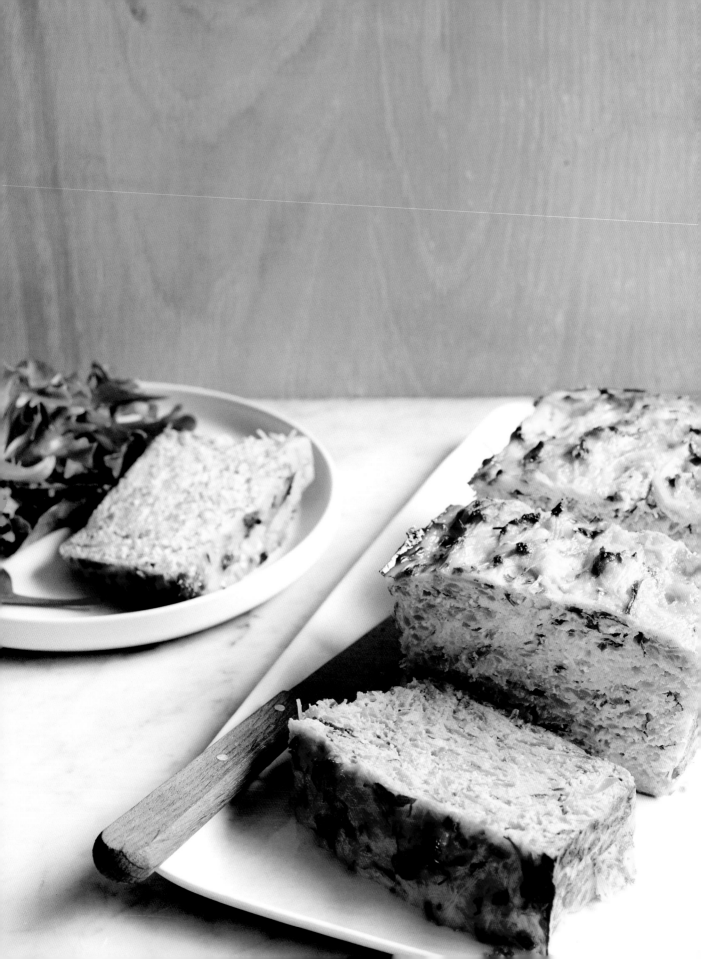

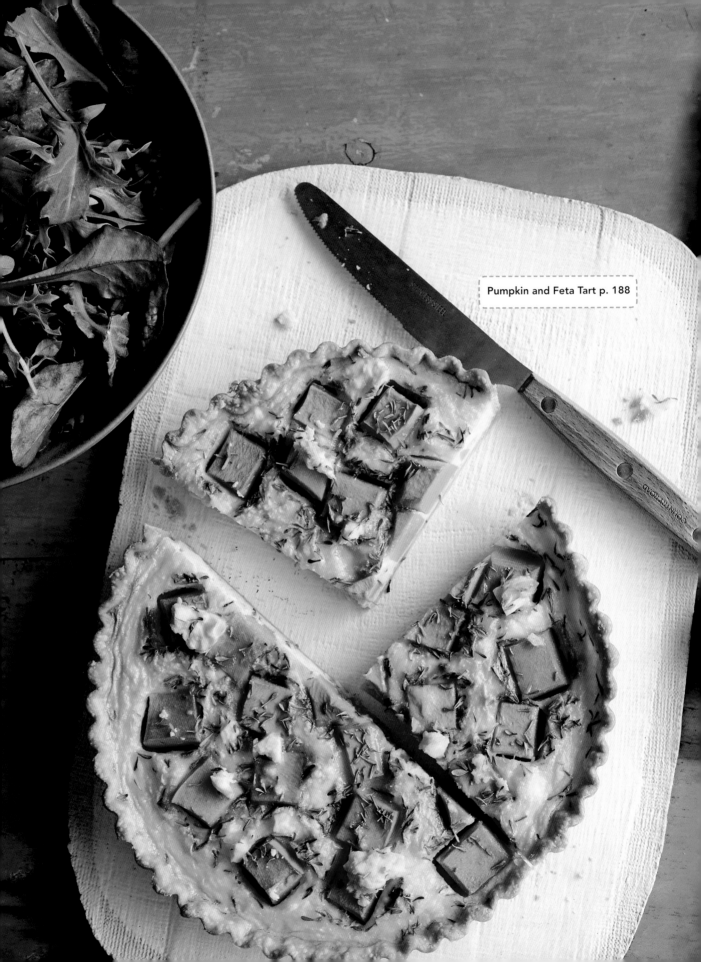

Pumpkin and Feta Tart p. 188

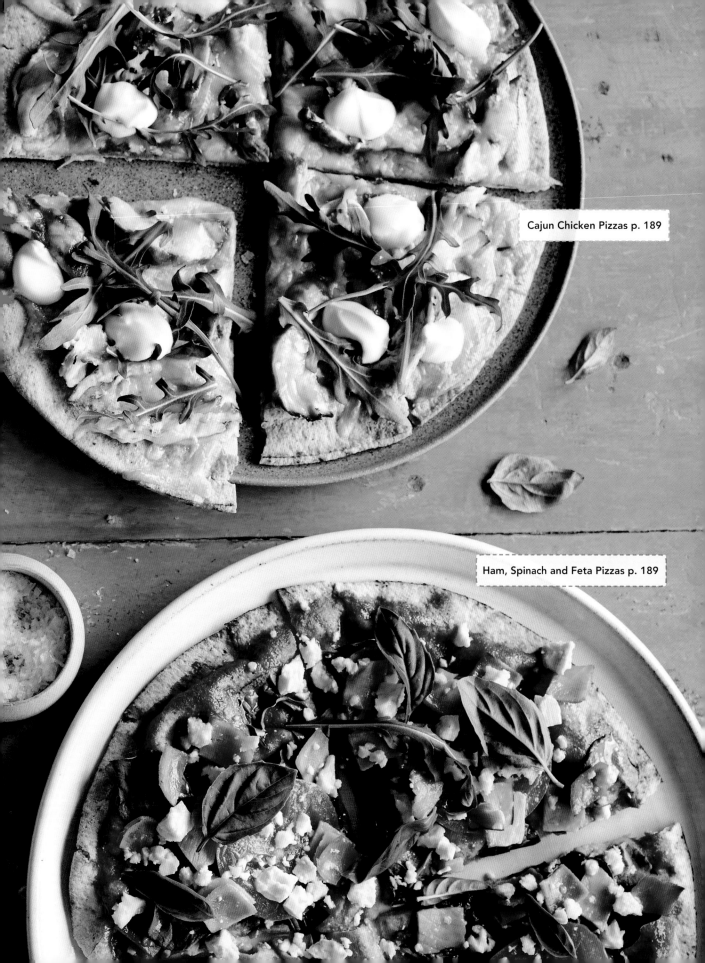

Cajun Chicken Pizzas p. 189

Ham, Spinach and Feta Pizzas p. 189

PUMPKIN AND FETA TART

SERVES
4

PREPARATION
15 MINS

COOK
45 MINS

COST PER SERVE
$1.15

cooking oil spray
1 sheet reduced-fat puff
  pastry, thawed
240 g pumpkin, peeled and
  seeds removed, cut into
  1 cm cubes
80 g reduced-fat feta,
  crumbled
1 teaspoon dried thyme
4 free-range eggs
¼ cup reduced-fat milk
  of choice
120 g mixed lettuce leaves

NUTRI DETAILS PER SERVE

1233 kJ/310 cals	Sat fat: 6.7 g
Protein: 16.4 g	Carbs: 23.4 g
Fibre: 4.2 g	Total sugar: 7.4 g
Total fat: 15.5 g	Free sugar: 0 g

Preheat the oven to 200°C.

Lightly spray a 20 cm tart tin with cooking oil and line with the pastry, pressing well into the side. Trim the edges, place on a baking tray and bake for 10–15 minutes until lightly golden. Set aside to cool.

Reduce the oven temperature to 170°C.

Arrange the pumpkin cubes over the pastry, then scatter over the feta and thyme.

Whisk the eggs and milk in a bowl. Pour the mixture over the pumpkin and bake for 30 minutes until the egg is set and the pumpkin is tender.

Cut into four even-sized pieces and serve with the mixed lettuce leaves on the side.

Store any leftovers in an airtight container in the fridge for 3–4 days or freeze for up to 2 months.

SUITABLE TO FREEZE

HAM, SPINACH AND FETA PIZZAS

SERVES	PREPARATION	COOK	COST PER SERVE
4	10 MINS	10 MINS	$2.50

4 medium wholemeal pita breads
1 cup tomato passata
120 g baby spinach leaves
2 tomatoes, sliced
8 slices lean smoked ham, diced
80 g reduced-fat feta
⅓ cup basil leaves

Preheat the oven to 200°C and line two baking trays with baking paper.

Place the pita breads on the prepared trays and spread evenly with the passata. Top with an even amount of spinach, tomato and ham.

Crumble the feta over the top and bake for 10 minutes until golden and crisp. Serve one pizza per person, sprinkled with the basil.

NUTRI DETAILS PER SERVE

1273 kJ/303 cals	Sat fat: 3 g
Protein: 20.1 g	Carbs: 36.4 g
Fibre: 7.1 g	Total sugar: 6.4 g
Total fat: 6.8 g	Free sugar: 0 g

CAJUN CHICKEN PIZZAS

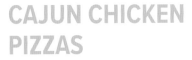

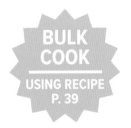

BULK COOK
USING RECIPE P. 39

SERVES	PREPARATION	COOK	COST PER SERVE
6	10 MINS	15 MINS, PLUS BASE RECIPE	$2.22

6 medium wholemeal pita breads
1 x quantity Cajun Chicken (see p. 39)
1½ cups grated reduced-fat cheddar
90 g rocket leaves
½ cup reduced-fat plain Greek yoghurt

Preheat the oven to 200°C and line two or three baking trays with baking paper.

Place the pita breads on the prepared trays and spread evenly with the Cajun chicken. Sprinkle over the grated cheese and bake for 10–15 minutes until the cheese has melted and the pita bread is crunchy.

Top each pizza with an even amount of rocket and 1 tablespoon yoghurt. Serve one pizza per person.

Store any leftover Cajun chicken in an airtight container in the fridge for 3–4 days or freeze for up to 2 months.

NUTRI DETAILS PER SERVE

1597 kJ/380 cals	Sat fat: 3.5 g
Protein: 36.4 g	Carbs: 35.4 g
Fibre: 9.1 g	Total sugar: 5.1 g
Total fat: 9.1 g	Free sugar: 0 g

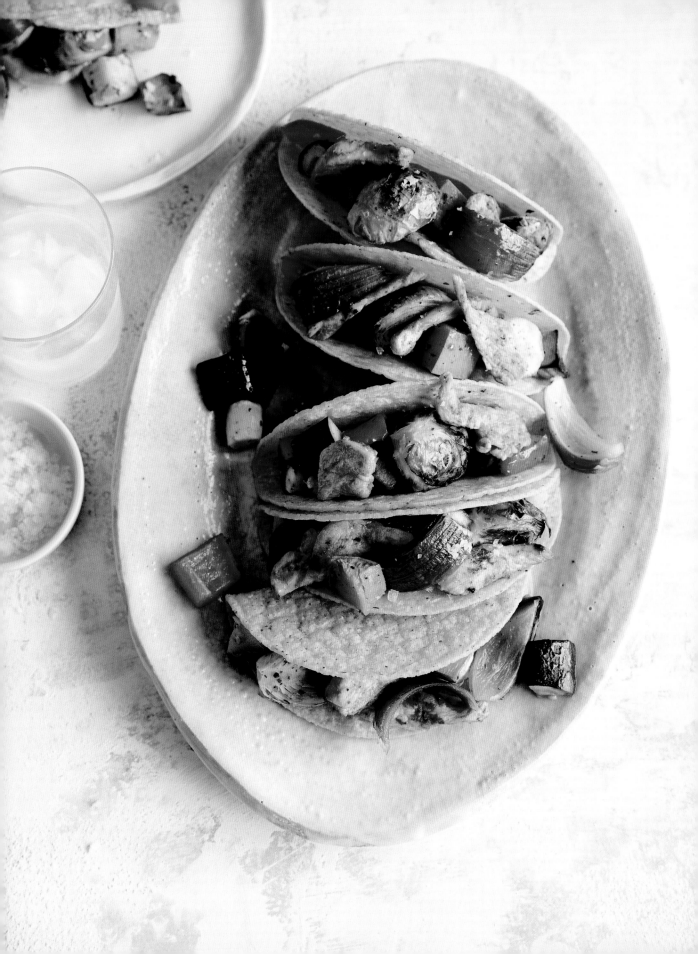

SPICED CHICKEN AND ROASTED RAINBOW VEGGIE TACOS

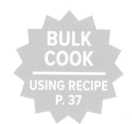

BULK COOK
USING RECIPE P. 37

SERVES
4

PREPARATION
10 MINS

COOK
10 MINS, PLUS
BASE RECIPE

COST PER SERVE
$2.50

1 x quantity Roasted Rainbow Veggies (see p. 37)
8 hard taco shells
240 g chicken breast fillet, thinly sliced
2 teaspoons red curry paste
cooking oil spray

NUTRI DETAILS PER SERVE

1829 kJ/435 cals
Protein: 22.7 g
Fibre: 9.8 g
Total fat: 18.7 g

Sat fat: 3.2 g
Carbs: 39.5 g
Total sugar: 17 g
Free sugar: 0 g

Reheat the roasted rainbow veggies in the microwave or on the stovetop until warmed through.

Heat the taco shells according to the packet directions.

Coat the chicken with the red curry paste.

Lightly spray a frying pan with cooking oil and heat over medium–high heat. Add the chicken and cook for 30–60 seconds each side until cooked through.

Fill each taco shell with roasted rainbow veggies and spiced chicken. Serve two filled tacos per person.

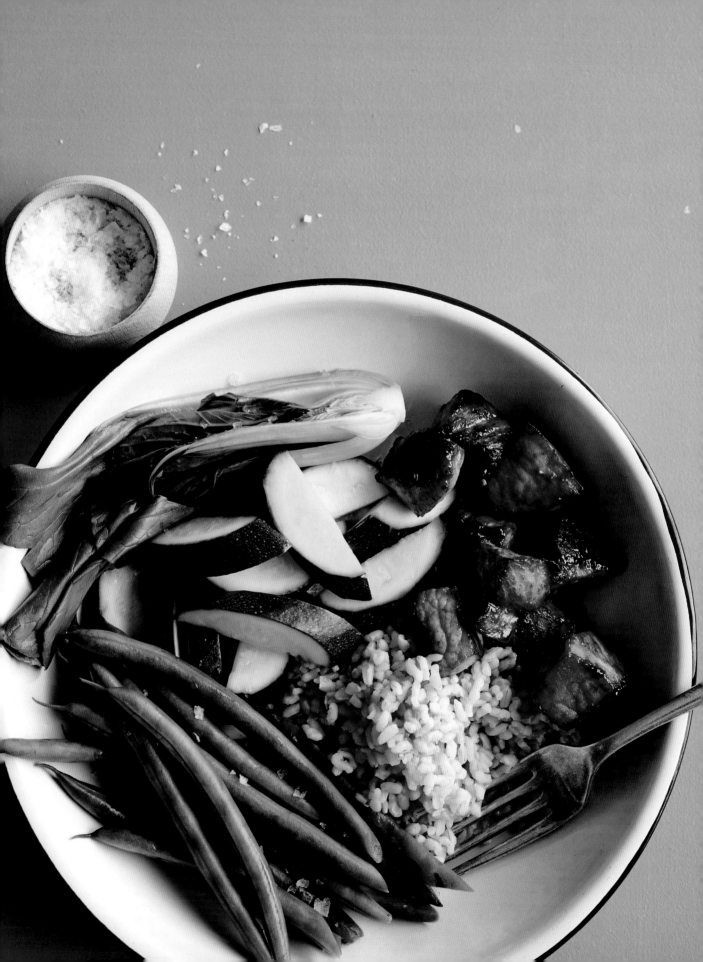

HOISIN PORK WITH GREENS AND RICE

SERVES
1

PREPARATION
10 MINS, PLUS
MARINATING TIME

COOK
25 MINS

COST PER SERVE
$2.50

1½ tablespoons brown rice
100 g pork loin fillet,
    trimmed and cut into
    bite-sized pieces
2 teaspoons hoisin sauce
½ small head bok choy,
    trimmed
60 g green beans, trimmed
½ small zucchini, sliced

NUTRI DETAILS PER SERVE

1040 kJ/248 cals	Sat fat: 1.8 g
Protein: 24.7 g	Carbs: 22 g
Fibre: 4.7 g	Total sugar: 5.6 g
Total fat: 5.6 g	Free sugar: 3.6 g

Preheat the oven to 200°C.

Bring 2 cups of water to the boil in a medium saucepan, add the rice and simmer for 25 minutes until tender. Drain. You could use pre-cooked rice for this recipe if you have some on hand. Just warm it through first.

Meanwhile, toss together the pork and hoisin sauce in a baking dish to coat. Set aside to marinate for 5 minutes (longer is better if you have time).

Place the marinated pork in the oven and bake for 10–15 minutes until cooked through.

While pork is cooking, steam the bok choy, beans and zucchini in the microwave or on the stovetop for about 5 minutes until tender crisp.

Serve the pork with the rice and greens on the side.

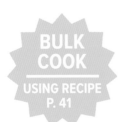
LAMB AND LENTIL
CURRY-STUFFED ZUCCHINI

SERVES
4

PREPARATION
10 MINS

COOK
30 MINS, PLUS
BASE RECIPE

COST PER SERVE
$2.50

---

4 small zucchini
cooking oil spray
1 x quantity Lamb and Lentil
   Curry (see p. 41)
pinch of salt

NUTRI DETAILS PER SERVE

1362 kJ/325 cals   Sat fat: 3.3 g
Protein: 27.8 g   Carbs: 22.2 g
Fibre: 9.6 g   Total sugar: 8.6 g
Total fat: 11.5 g   Free sugar: 0 g

FOR A VEGETARIAN MEAL

Omit the lamb, use vegetable stock
and add 320 g diced sweet potato
and a drained 400 g can of corn kernels
to the curry.

COST PER SERVE $2.07

Preheat the oven to 200°C and line a baking tray with baking paper.

Cut the zucchini in half lengthways and place on the prepared tray, cut-side down. Spray with cooking oil and bake for 10 minutes.

Meanwhile, reheat the lamb and lentil curry in the microwave or on the stovetop until warmed through.

Remove the zucchini from the oven and scoop out some of the flesh, leaving a shell strong enough to hold the filling. Dice the flesh and mix through the lamb and lentil curry.

Spoon the lamb mixture evenly into the zucchini halves. Return to the oven and bake for another 15–20 minutes until the zucchini shells are tender and the lamb filling is bubbling. Sprinkle with salt and serve. Two stuffed zucchini halves is one serve.

Store any leftover curry in an airtight container in the fridge for 4–5 days or freeze for up to 3 months.

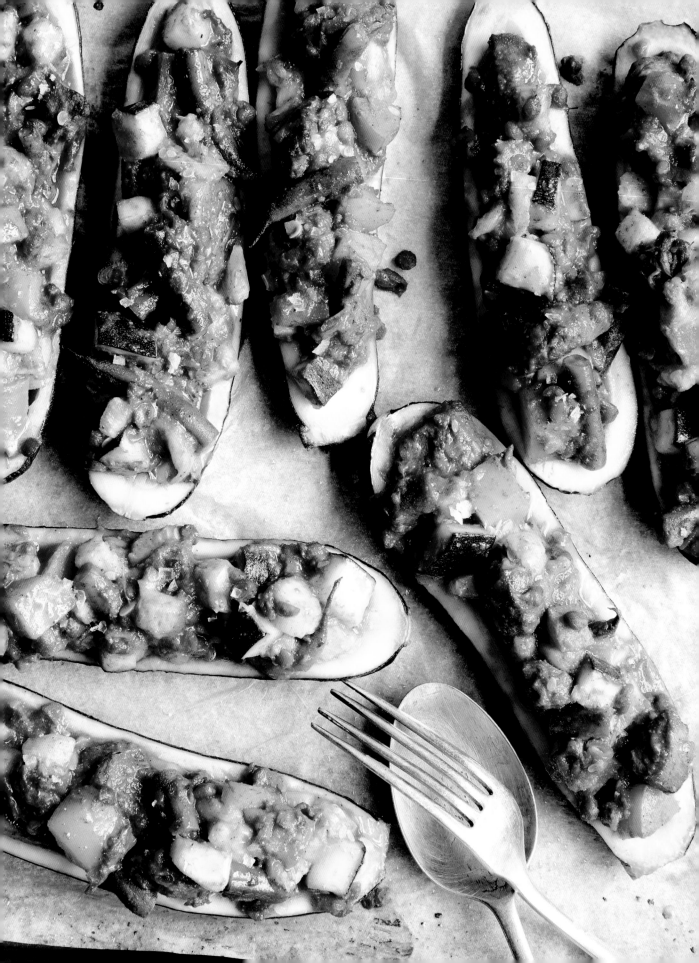

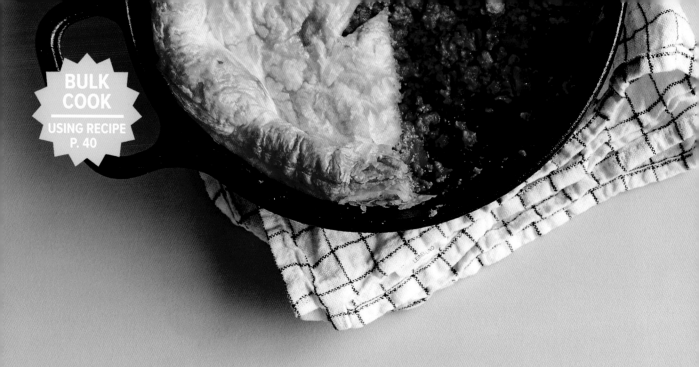

BULK COOK

USING RECIPE P. 40

HIDDEN VEG BOLOGNESE PIE

SERVES
4

PREPARATION
10 MINS

COOK
30 MINS, PLUS
BASE RECIPE

COST PER SERVE
$1.22

---

1 x quantity **Hidden Veg Bolognese** (see p. 40)
1 sheet **reduced-fat puff pastry**, thawed
1 tablespoon **milk of choice**

NUTRI DETAILS PER SERVE

1457 kJ/347 cals	Sat fat: 7 g
Protein: 21.5 g	Carbs: 24.2 g
Fibre: 3.2 g	Total sugar: 5.9 g
Total fat: 17.6 g	Free sugar: 0 g

FOR A VEGETARIAN MEAL

Use vegetable stock and replace the mince with 2 × 400 g cans of lentils, drained and rinsed.

COST PER SERVE $1.00

Preheat the oven to 180°C.

Reheat the hidden veg bolognese in the microwave or on the stovetop until warmed through.

Transfer the meat sauce to a baking dish and cover with the puff pastry sheet, trimming the edges to fit the dish. Brush the pastry with the milk and pierce with a knife in the centre, to allow the steam to escape during cooking.

Bake for 20 minutes until the pastry is golden and crisp.

Cut into four even-sized pieces and serve.

Store any leftovers in an airtight container in the fridge for 2–3 days or freeze for up to 3 months.

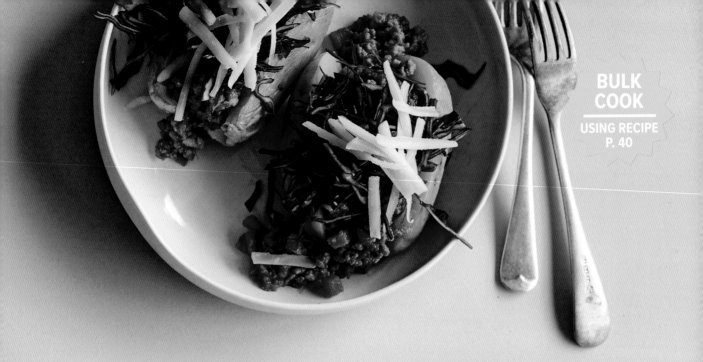

BULK COOK

USING RECIPE P. 40

HIDDEN VEG BOLOGNESE POTATOES

SERVES
4

PREPARATION
10 MINS

COOK
20 MINS, PLUS
BASE RECIPE

COST PER SERVE
$1.80

---

4 potatoes (about 120 g each)
1 x quantity Hidden Veg
Bolognese (see p. 40)
100 g red cabbage, shredded
⅔ cup grated reduced-fat
cheddar

NUTRI DETAILS PER SERVE

1612 kJ/383 cals   Sat fat: 5.6 g
Protein: 35.3 g   Carbs: 21 g
Fibre: 5.7 g   Total sugar: 5.7 g
Total fat: 16.2 g   Free sugar: 0 g

FOR A VEGETARIAN MEAL

Use vegetable stock and replace the
mince with 2 × 400 g cans lentils,
drained and rinsed.

COST PER SERVE $1.57

Place the potatoes in a saucepan of water and bring to the boil.
Cook for 15–20 minutes until soft.

Meanwhile, reheat the hidden veg bolognese in the microwave
or on the stovetop until warmed through.

Cut each potato down the centre and gently pull apart (like you
would a jacket potato). Fill with an even amount of the hidden veg
bolognese. Sprinkle over the shredded cabbage and grated cheese
and serve.

Store any leftover bolognese in an airtight container in the fridge
for 2–3 days or freeze for up to 3 months.

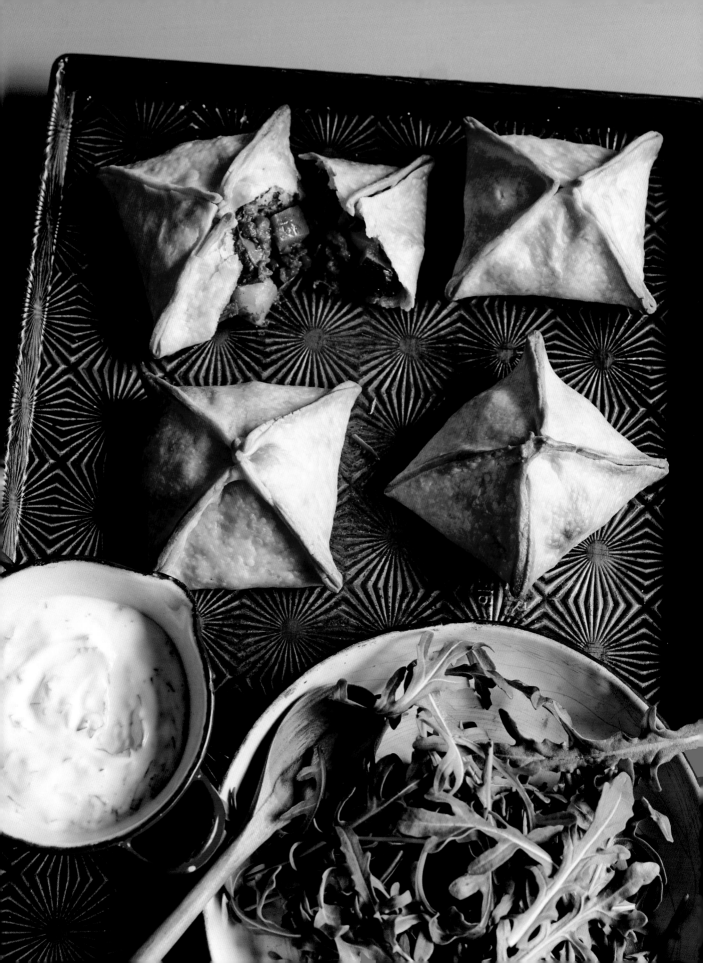

LAMB AND LENTIL CURRY PASTIES

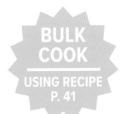
BULK COOK
USING RECIPE P. 41

SERVES
4

PREPARATION
10 MINS

COOK
40 MINS, PLUS
BASE RECIPE

COST PER SERVE
$1.24

1 sheet reduced-fat puff
pastry, thawed
⅓ x quantity Lamb and Lentil
Curry (see p. 41)
2 tablespoons reduced-fat
milk of choice
⅓ cup reduced-fat plain
Greek yoghurt
1 tablespoon chopped
mint leaves
freshly ground black pepper
30 g rocket leaves

NUTRI DETAILS PER SERVE

1906 kJ/ 454 cals	Sat fat: 5.7 g
Protein: 31.3 g	Carbs: 40.7 g
Fibre: 16.3 g	Total sugar: 9.2 g
Total fat: 9.5 g	Free sugar: 0 g

FOR A VEGETARIAN MEAL

Omit the lamb, use vegetable stock
and add 320 g diced sweet potato
and a drained 400 g can of corn kernels
to the curry.

COST PER SERVE $0.95

Preheat the oven to 200°C and line a baking tray with baking paper.

Cut the pastry into four even squares. Place an even amount of the lamb and lentil curry in the middle of each pastry square. Fold in the pastry corners so they meet in the middle and pinch them together. Brush with a little milk and place on the prepared tray.

Bake for 20–30 minutes until the pastry is crisp and golden.

Meanwhile, combine the yoghurt and mint in a bowl and season with pepper.

Divide the rocket leaves evenly among four plates. Top with a lamb and lentil curry pasty and a dollop of mint yoghurt and serve.

Store any leftover pasties in an airtight container in the fridge for 4–5 days or freeze for up to 2 months.

SLOW-COOKED BEEF NACHOS

SERVES
10

PREPARATION
15 MINS

COOK
8 HOURS
10 MINS

COST PER SERVE
$2.25

1.1 kg beef rolled roast
1 brown onion, diced
2 garlic cloves, crushed
1 × 400 g can red kidney
   beans, drained and rinsed
1 × 400 g can diced tomatoes
1 tablespoon sliced pickled
   jalapeno chilli
1 green capsicum, diced
2 teaspoons chilli powder
1 teaspoon smoked paprika
1 teaspoon onion powder
½ teaspoon ground cumin
200 g plain corn chips
2 cups grated reduced-fat
   cheddar

NUTRI DETAILS PER SERVE

1502 kJ/358 cals	Sat fat: 5.7 g
Protein: 38.2 g	Carbs: 18.3 g
Fibre: 5.5 g	Total sugar: 3.3 g
Total fat: 13.4 g	Free sugar: 0 g

If cooking in the oven:
Preheat the oven to 120°C.

Place the beef, onion, garlic, kidney beans, tomatoes, jalapeno, capsicum, chilli powder, paprika, onion powder and cumin in a large casserole dish. Stir well to combine and cover with the lid.

Bake for at least 8 hours until the beef is falling apart and very tender. Add some water if the beef starts to dry out at any stage.

Remove the beef from the dish. Using two forks, shred the meat into small pieces, then return to the sauce in the dish.

If cooking in a slow cooker:
Place the beef, onion, garlic, kidney beans, tomatoes, jalapeno, capsicum, chilli powder, paprika, onion powder, cumin and 2 cups of water in the slow cooker dish. Stir well to combine and cover with the lid.

Cook on low for 8 hours until the beef is falling apart and very tender. Add more water during cooking if the meat starts to dry out.

Remove the beef from the dish. Using two forks, shred the meat into small pieces, then return to the sauce in the dish.

To serve:
Preheat the oven to 180°C.

Arrange the corn chips on one large dish for everyone to share or divide them evenly among 10 small ovenproof dishes. Top with the chilli beef and sprinkle with the cheese.

Bake for 5–10 minutes until the cheese has melted. Serve, being careful of the hot serving dishes.

Store any leftover beef in an airtight container in the fridge for 4–5 days or freeze for up to 4 months.

SLOW-COOKED BEEF IS SUITABLE TO FREEZE

You could serve this with a dollop of reduced-fat plain Greek yoghurt or extra-light sour cream, if you like.

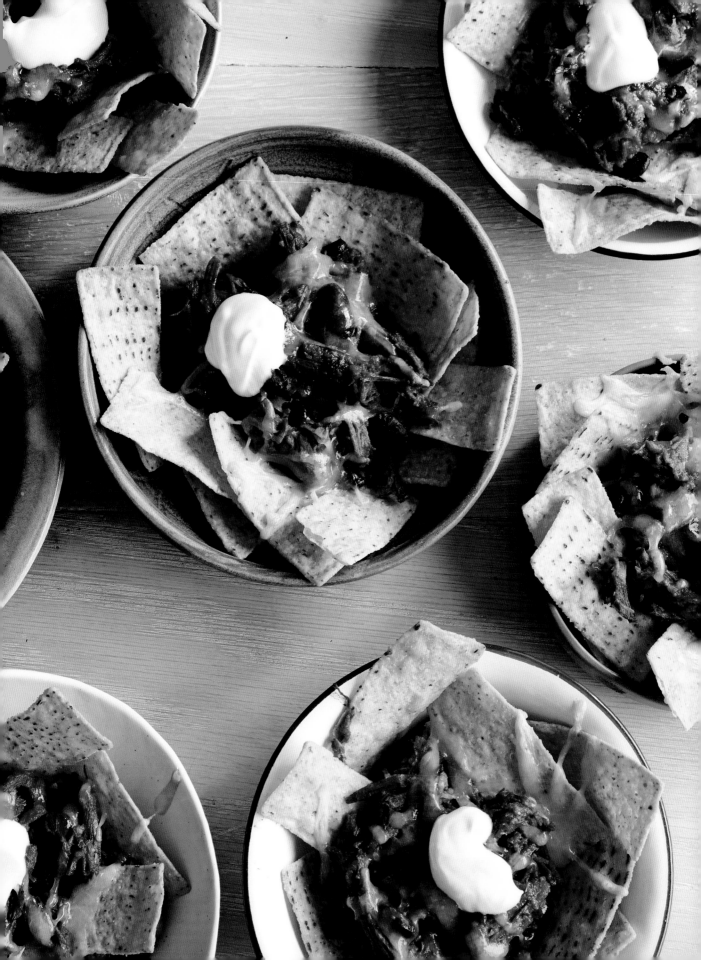

SNACKS

Healthy hunger-beaters!

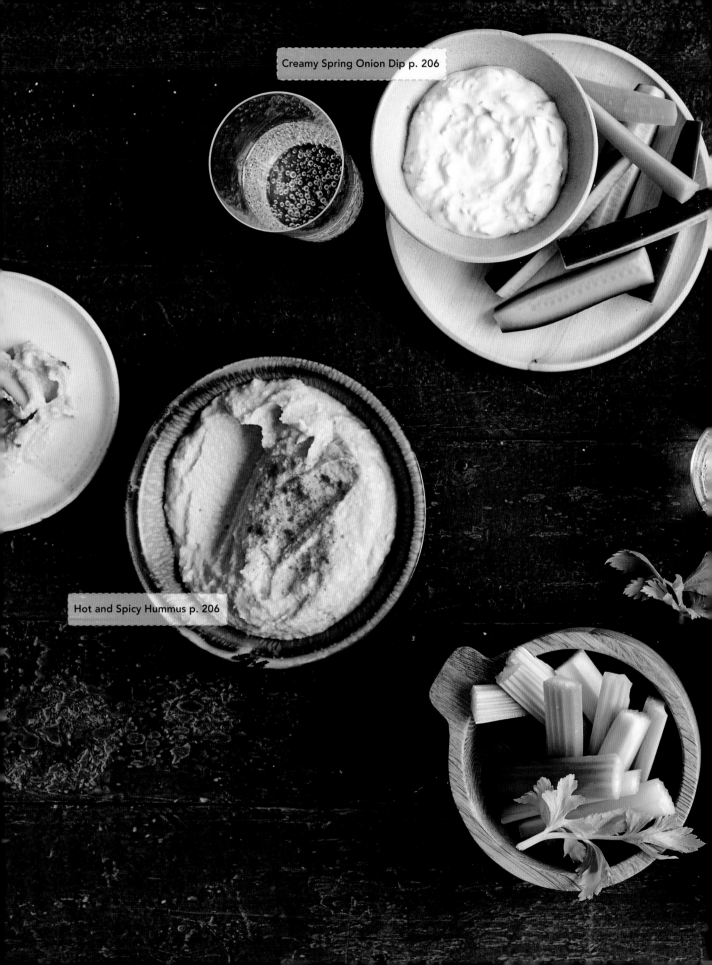

Creamy Spring Onion Dip p. 206

Hot and Spicy Hummus p. 206

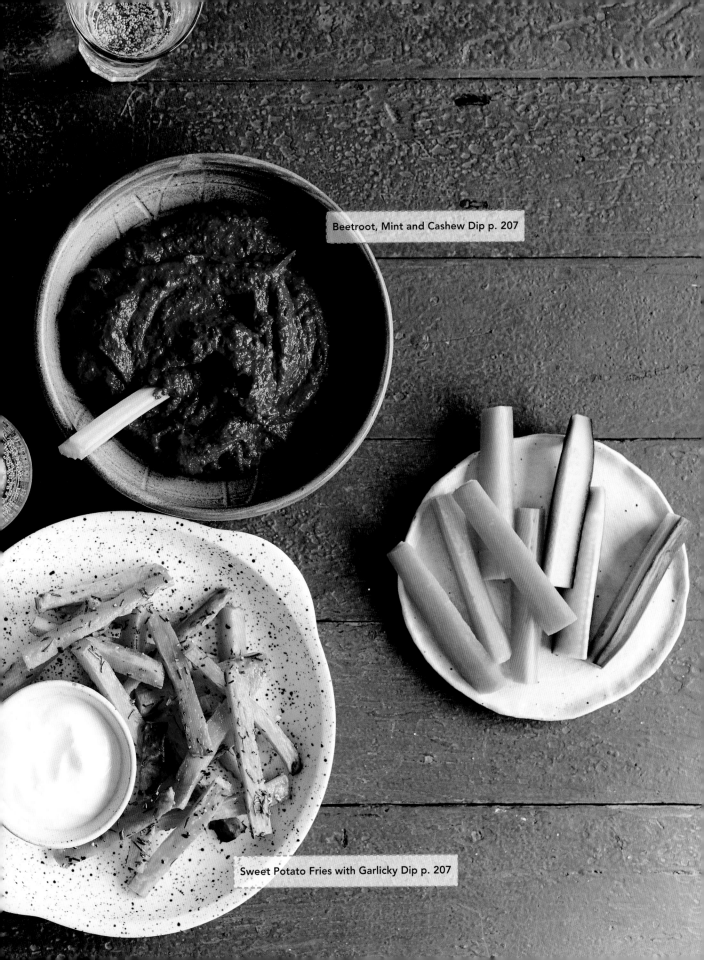

Beetroot, Mint and Cashew Dip p. 207

Sweet Potato Fries with Garlicky Dip p. 207

CREAMY SPRING ONION DIP

SERVES
1

PREPARATION
5 MINS

COST PER SERVE
$0.54

1 spring onion, finely diced
¼ garlic clove, crushed
1 tablespoon light cream cheese
¼ cup reduced-fat plain Greek yoghurt
1 carrot, sliced into batons

Combine the spring onion, garlic, cream cheese and yoghurt in a bowl. Serve with the carrot dippers.

NUTRI DETAILS PER SERVE

458 kJ/109 cals	Sat fat: 2.9 g
Protein: 5.7 g	Carbs: 9.8 g
Fibre: 2.5 g	Total sugar: 9.6 g
Total fat: 4.5 g	Free sugar: 0 g

HOT AND SPICY HUMMUS

SERVES
4

PREPARATION
10 MINS

COST PER SERVE
$0.68

1 × 400 g can chickpeas, drained and rinsed
2 garlic cloves
pinch of salt
¼ teaspoon cayenne pepper
¼ teaspoon chilli powder
¼ teaspoon smoked paprika
2 tablespoons extra-virgin olive oil
1 tablespoon tahini
¼ cup lemon juice
2 carrots (or 2 celery stalks), sliced into batons
1 Lebanese cucumber, sliced into batons

Place the chickpeas, garlic, salt, spices, olive oil, tahini and lemon juice in a food processor and blitz until smooth. Add a little water to thin it down, if required.

Serve the hummus with the vegetable dippers.

Store any leftover hummus in an airtight container in the fridge for 4–5 days.

NUTRI DETAILS PER SERVE

993 kJ/236 cals	Sat fat: 1.8 g
Protein: 7.8 g	Carbs: 17 g
Fibre: 7 g	Total sugar: 4 g
Total fat: 14 g	Free sugar: 0 g

BEETROOT, MINT AND CASHEW DIP

SERVES
4

PREPARATION
10 MINS, PLUS
COOLING TIME

COOK
20 MINS

COST PER SERVE
$1.03

4 small beetroot, peeled and chopped
⅓ cup reduced-fat plain Greek yoghurt
⅓ cup unsalted cashews
1 tablespoon lemon juice
1 tablespoon extra-virgin olive oil
⅓ cup mint leaves
salt and freshly ground black pepper
4 carrots, sliced into batons

Steam the beetroot in the microwave or on the stovetop for 20 minutes until very tender. Set aside to cool.

Place the beetroot, yoghurt, cashews, lemon juice, olive oil and mint in a food processor. Season with salt and pepper and blitz until smooth.

Serve the dip with the vegetable dippers.

Store any leftover dip in an airtight container in the fridge for 4–5 days.

NUTRI DETAILS PER SERVE

625 kJ/149 cals	Sat fat: 1.4 g
Protein: 3.9 g	Carbs: 12.9 g
Fibre: 5.4 g	Total sugar: 11.9 g
Total fat: 8 g	Free sugar: 0 g

SWEET POTATO FRIES WITH GARLICKY DIP

SERVES
1

PREPARATION
10 MINS

COOK
15 MINS

COST PER SERVE
$1.19

½ small sweet potato
1 teaspoon extra-virgin olive oil
1 tablespoon chopped rosemary leaves
salt and freshly ground black pepper
½ garlic clove, crushed
¼ cup reduced-fat plain Greek yoghurt
1 teaspoon lemon juice

Preheat the oven to 200°C and line a baking tray with baking paper.

Slice the sweet potato into thin chips (a bit thicker than French fries). Toss with the olive oil and rosemary to coat and season with a little salt and pepper.

Spread the fries over the prepared tray in a single layer and roast for 15 minutes until tender inside and crunchy outside.

Meanwhile, combine the garlic, yoghurt and lemon juice in a bowl and season to taste with salt and pepper.

Serve the fries with the garlicky dip on the side.

NUTRI DETAILS PER SERVE

638 kJ/152 cals	Sat fat: 5.5 g
Protein: 5 g	Carbs: 17.2 g
Fibre: 2 g	Total sugar: 9.8 g
Total fat: 6.2 g	Free sugar: 0 g

SPICY BROCCOLI AND CHEESE PIKELETS

SERVES
3

PREPARATION
10 MINS

COOK
5 MINS

COST PER SERVE
$0.38

½ cup wholemeal plain flour
1 teaspoon baking powder
1 free-range egg
¼ cup reduced-fat milk
   of choice
25 g broccoli, finely chopped
¼ cup grated reduced-fat
   cheddar
½ teaspoon dried chilli flakes
salt and freshly ground
   black pepper
1 teaspoon extra-virgin
   olive oil

NUTRI DETAILS PER SERVE

657 kJ/156 cals	Sat fat: 3.2 g
Protein: 8.6 g	Carbs: 18.3 g
Fibre: 1.2 g	Total sugar: 1.2 g
Total fat: 5.2 g	Free sugar: 0 g

Whisk the flour, baking powder, egg and milk to form a batter. Stir in the broccoli and cheddar. Sprinkle in the chilli flakes and season with salt and pepper, then stir to combine.

Heat the olive oil in a large frying pan over medium–high heat. Spoon tablespoons of the batter into the pan to make nine pikelets in total (depending on the size of your pan, you may need to cook them in batches). Cook for 1–2 minutes on each side until golden. Three pikelets is one serve.

Store any leftovers in an airtight container in the fridge for 3–4 days or freeze for up to 2 months.

SUITABLE TO FREEZE

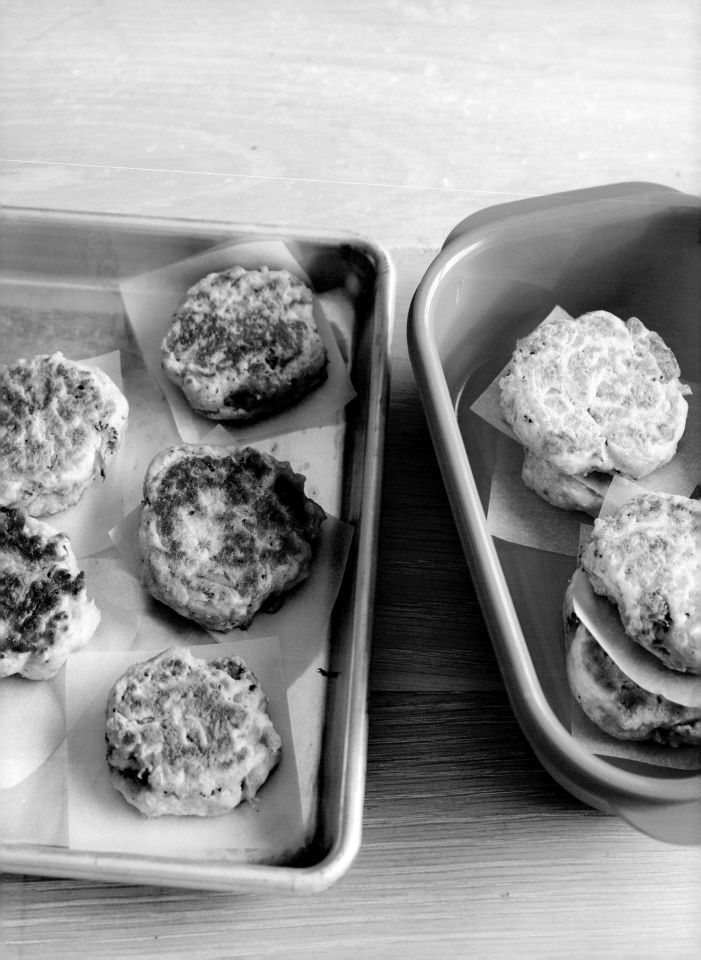

CHEESE AND OLIVE PINWHEELS

SERVES
6

PREPARATION
10 MINS

COOK
20 MINS

COST PER SERVE
$0.33

---

1 garlic clove
1 tablespoon dried rosemary
1 cup pitted kalamata olives
1 sheet reduced-fat puff
  pastry, thawed
½ cup grated reduced-fat
  cheddar

NUTRI DETAILS PER SERVE

684 kJ/163 cals	Sat fat: 2 g
Protein: 5 g	Carbs: 16 g
Fibre: 1 g	Total sugar: 6 g
Total fat: 9 g	Free sugar: 0 g

Preheat the oven to 200°C and line a baking tray with baking paper.

Place the garlic, rosemary and olives in a blender or small food processor and pulse to form a chunky paste.

Spread the olive paste over the pastry sheet and sprinkle evenly with the cheddar. Roll up the pastry to form a log, then carefully slice into 12 even-sized pieces.

Place the pinwheels on the prepared tray and bake for 15–20 minutes until the pastry is cooked through and golden. Two pinwheels is one serve.

Store any leftovers in an airtight container in the fridge for 3–4 days or freeze for up to 3 months.

SUITABLE TO FREEZE

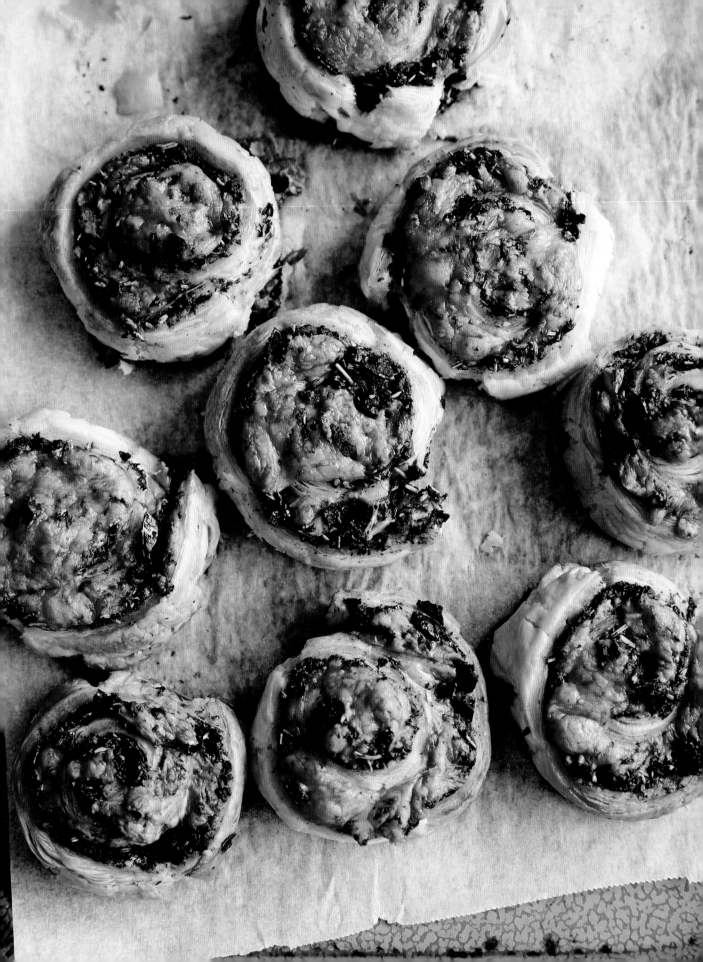

MINI CHEESE, HAM AND QUINOA MUFFINS

SERVES
6

PREPARATION
10 MINS, PLUS
COOLING TIME

COOK
35 MINS

COST PER SERVE
$0.40

cooking oil spray (optional)
¼ cup quinoa, rinsed
2 slices lean smoked ham, diced
1 free-range egg
1 free-range egg white
½ large zucchini, grated
½ cup grated reduced-fat cheddar
1½ tablespoons grated parmesan

NUTRI DETAILS PER SERVE

282 kJ/67 cals	Sat fat: 1.2 g
Protein: 6.3 g	Carbs: 4.4 g
Fibre: 0.6 g	Total sugar: 1 g
Total fat: 2.6 g	Free sugar: 0 g

Preheat the oven to 180°C. Line or lightly grease 12 holes of a mini muffin tin.

Place the quinoa and ½ cup of water in a small saucepan and bring to the boil. Reduce the heat and simmer, covered, for 15 minutes until tender and most of the liquid has been absorbed. Fluff up with a fork, then set aside to cool slightly.

Place the cooled quinoa in a bowl, add the remaining ingredients and mix well to combine. Divide the batter evenly among the prepared muffin holes.

Bake for 15 minutes until golden and a skewer inserted into the centre of a muffin comes out clean. Cool in the tin for 5 minutes before turning out onto a wire rack. Two mini muffins is one serve.

Store any leftover cooled muffins in an airtight container in the fridge for 3–4 days or freeze for up to 2 months.

SUITABLE TO FREEZE

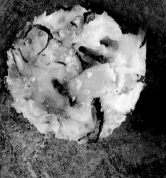
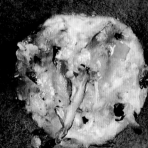

ASPARAGUS AND CHICKEN MINI QUICHES

SERVES
6

PREPARATION
15 MINS, PLUS
COOLING TIME

COOK
15 MINS

COST PER SERVE
$1.90

cooking oil spray
300 g chicken breast fillet
salt and freshly ground
   black pepper
3 wholemeal mountain
   bread wraps
1½ garlic cloves, grated
6 asparagus spears, woody
   ends trimmed, diced
12 free-range eggs, beaten

NUTRI DETAILS PER SERVE

849 kJ/203 cals	Sat fat: 3 g
Protein: 20 g	Carbs: 9 g
Fibre: 2 g	Total sugar: 1 g
Total fat: 10 g	Free sugar: 0 g

Preheat the oven to 180°C and generously grease 12 holes of a standard muffin tin.

Lightly spray a frying pan with cooking oil. Season the chicken with salt and pepper, then add to the pan and cook for 2–3 minutes on each side until cooked through. Set aside to cool, then shred the meat with two forks. You could use pre-cooked or leftover chicken for this recipe if you have some on hand.

Cut the mountain bread wraps into quarters. Line each muffin hole with a piece of bread to form the base for the quiches.

Place the chicken, garlic and asparagus in a bowl. Season with salt and pepper and mix well.

Spoon the chicken mixture evenly into the lined muffin holes and then pour the egg over the filling. Bake for 10–12 minutes until the egg has set. Two quiches is one serve.

Store any leftovers in an airtight container in the fridge for 3–4 days or freeze for up to 2 months.

SUITABLE TO FREEZE

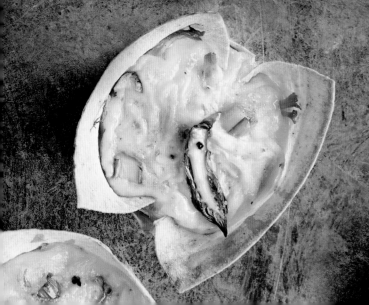

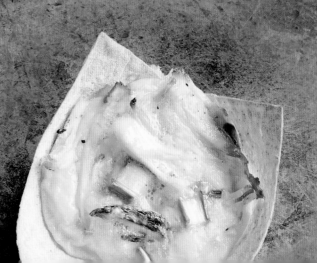

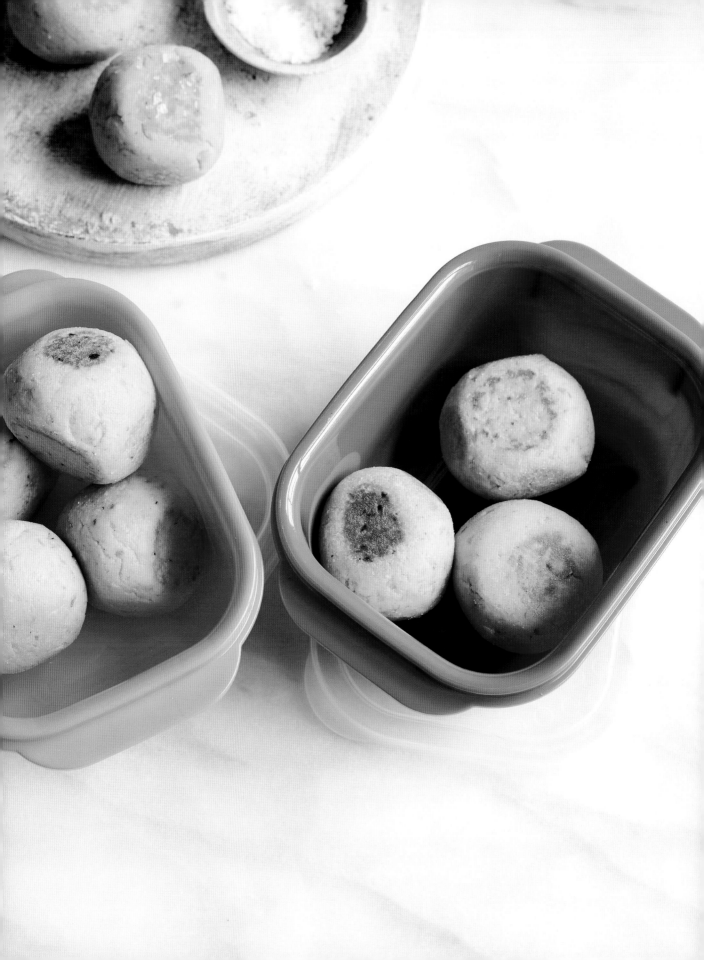

CAJUN CHICKEN MEATBALLS

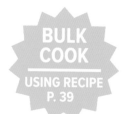

BULK COOK

USING RECIPE P. 39

SERVES
6

PREPARATION
15 MINS

COOK
15 MINS, PLUS
BASE RECIPE

COST PER SERVE
$1.20

1 x quantity Cajun Chicken
(see p. 39), cold
3 teaspoons grated parmesan
3 free-range eggs
1½ carrots, grated
¾ cup rice flour
cooking oil spray (optional)

NUTRI DETAILS PER SERVE

700 kJ/167 cals	Sat fat: 1.6 g
Protein: 13.8 g	Carbs: 16.5 g
Fibre: 1.4 g	Total sugar: 0.9 g
Total fat: 5.3 g	Free sugar: 0 g

Preheat the oven to 200°C and line a baking tray with baking paper.

Place the Cajun chicken in a food processor with the parmesan and eggs and blitz until combined. Add the carrot and blitz until just incorporated.

Gradually add the rice flour until the mixture forms a soft dough that sticks together. You may not need to use all the flour – it depends on the consistency of the Cajun chicken (if it's really moist, use more flour; if it's drier, use less flour).

Roll the mixture into 18 balls and place on the prepared tray. Bake for 10–15 minutes until golden brown. You could also pan-fry the meatballs like fritters if preferred; spray a large frying pan with cooking oil and cook the meatballs over medium–high heat, turning frequently, until golden all over. Three meatballs is one serve.

Store any leftover meatballs in the fridge for 3–4 days or freeze for up to 2 months.

ASIAN PORK AND VEGGIE RICE BALLS

SERVES
4

PREPARATION
10 MINS, PLUS
COOLING TIME

COOK
35 MINS

COST PER SERVE
$0.71

½ cup basmati rice
1 spring onion, finely sliced
1 celery stalk, finely diced
1 carrot, grated
1 free-range egg white,
  lightly beaten
1 tablespoon black or
  white sesame seeds
2 teaspoons tamari
  (gluten-free soy sauce)
150 g lean pork mince
cooking oil spray

NUTRI DETAILS PER SERVE

718 kJ/171 cals	Sat fat: 1.2 g
Protein: 11 g	Carbs: 21.4 g
Fibre: 1 g	Total sugar: 1 g
Total fat: 4.3 g	Free sugar: 0 g

Preheat the oven to 180°C and line a baking tray with baking paper.

Bring 2 cups of water to the boil in a small saucepan, add the rice and simmer for 10–12 minutes or until tender. Drain and set aside to cool.

Place the cooled rice, spring onion, celery, carrot, egg white, sesame seeds, tamari and pork mince in a bowl and mix well with your hands. Form the mixture into 12 balls and place on the prepared tray.

Lightly spray the balls with cooking oil and bake for 20 minutes until golden and cooked through. Three balls is one serve.

Store any leftover balls in an airtight container in the fridge for 3–4 days to reheat or enjoy cold, or freeze for up to 2 months.

SUITABLE TO FREEZE

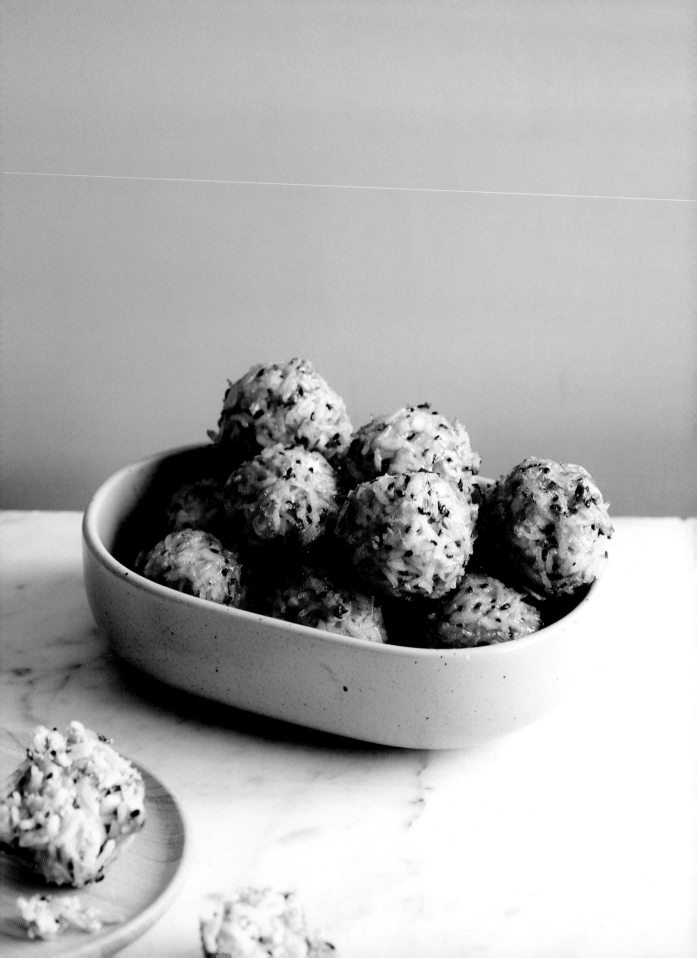

SWEETS
& DESSERTS

Because we all need a treat!

CHOC–MARSHMALLOW SLICE

SERVES
24

PREPARATION
45 MINS, PLUS
FREEZING TIME

COST PER SERVE
$0.56

½ cup cacao powder
½ cup coconut oil
½ teaspoon liquid stevia

BISCUIT BASE
1 cup medjool dates, pitted
½ cup coconut oil
2 teaspoons vanilla extract
2 ¼ cups oat bran
½ cup coconut flour

MARSHMALLOW LAYER
3 tablespoons powdered
   gelatine
½ cup warm water
1 cup boiling water
1½ tablespoons stevia
   powder
½ teaspoon vanilla extract
270 ml reduced-fat
   coconut milk

NUTRI DETAILS PER SERVE

784 kJ/187 cals	Sat fat: 7.1 g
Protein: 4.2 g	Carbs: 13 g
Fibre: 2.5 g	Total sugar: 5.4 g
Total fat: 12.6 g	Free sugar: 0 g

Line a 20 cm x 30 cm slice tin with baking paper.

To make the biscuit base, place the dates, coconut oil, vanilla, oat bran, coconut flour and ¼ cup of water in a food processor and blitz briefly to combine. Press the mixture evenly into the base of the prepared tin, then freeze for 15–20 minutes until set.

Meanwhile, to make the marshmallow layer, dissolve the powdered gelatine in the ½ cup of warm water and whisk for 5 minutes until it becomes gel-like.

Mix the 1 cup of boiling water with the stevia and vanilla, stirring until the stevia has dissolved. Add to the gelatine mixture with the coconut milk and whisk with electric beaters for 10 minutes, until smooth and thick. Pour over the biscuit base and return to the freezer for another 20 minutes until the marshmallow is set.

Shortly before the marshmallow layer is ready, place the cacao powder and coconut oil in a small saucepan and stir over low heat until melted and combined. Stir in the liquid stevia.

Pour the chocolate over the marshmallow layer and smooth the surface with the back of a spoon. Place the slice in the freezer for another 20 minutes to set the chocolate layer.

When set, remove the slice from the tin and allow to sit on the bench for 5–10 minutes, then, using a knife dipped in boiling water, cut into 24 bite-sized squares. One square is one serve.

Store any leftovers in an airtight container in the fridge for up to 1 week or freeze for 1 month.

SUITABLE TO FREEZE

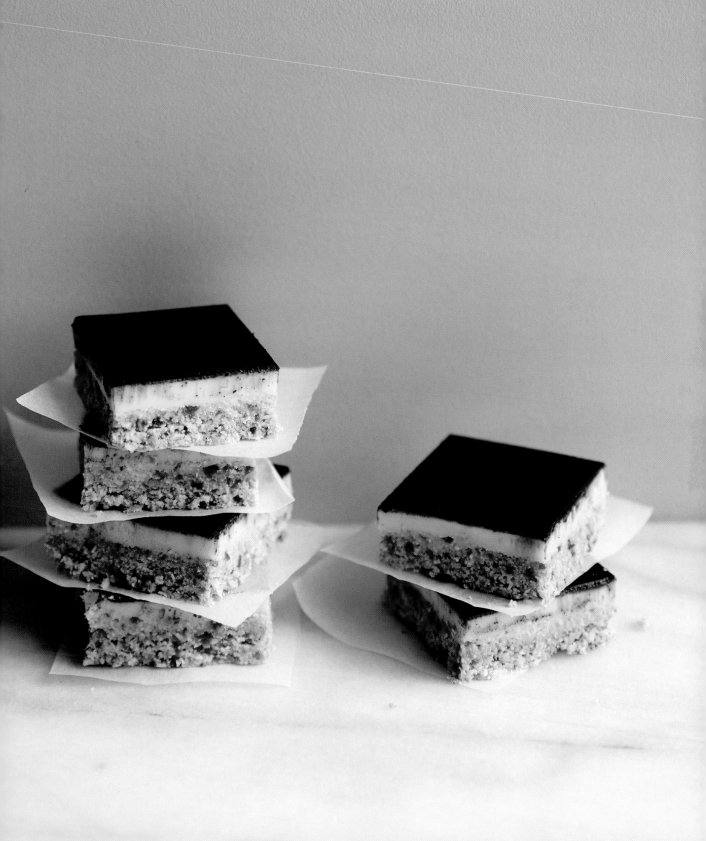

COCONUT–DATE LOAF

SERVES
10

PREPARATION
10 MINS, PLUS
COOLING TIME

COOK
35 MINS

COST PER SERVE
$0.35

---

1 cup pitted dates,
  chopped
1½ cups wholemeal self-
  raising flour
¼ cup coconut sugar
⅓ cup desiccated coconut
½ teaspoon bicarbonate
  of soda
½ teaspoon ground cinnamon
½ cup reduced-fat milk
  of choice
60 g butter, melted
2 free-range eggs
1 teaspoon vanilla extract

NUTRI DETAILS PER SERVE

917 kJ/218 cals	Sat fat: 5.3 g
Protein: 4.7 g	Carbs: 29 g
Fibre: 4.3 g	Total sugar: 17 g
Total fat: 8.4 g	Free sugar: 4.7 g

Preheat the oven to 180°C and line a standard loaf tin with baking paper.

Combine the dates, flour, coconut sugar, desiccated coconut, bicarbonate of soda and cinnamon in a bowl. Add the milk, butter, eggs and vanilla and mix to combine. Pour the mixture into the prepared tin and smooth the surface.

Bake for 30–35 minutes until a skewer inserted into the centre of the loaf comes out clean. Remove from the oven and cool in the tin for 5 minutes, then turn out onto a wire rack to cool completely.

Slice into 10 even-sized pieces. One piece is one serve.

Store any leftovers in an airtight container in the fridge for 3–4 days or freeze individual slices for up to 2 months.

SUITABLE TO FREEZE

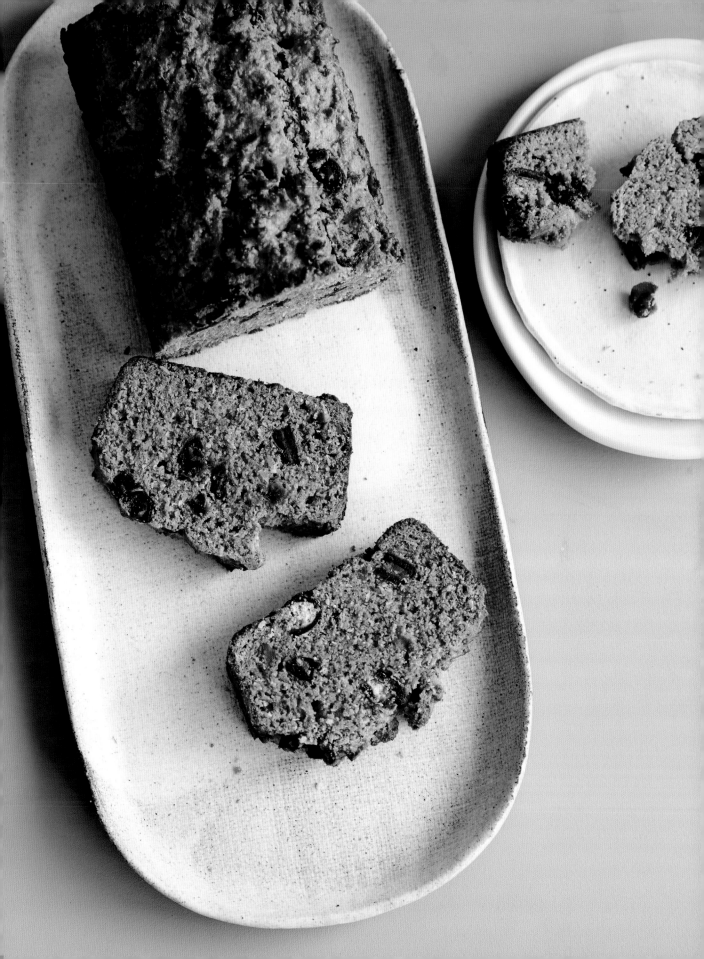

APRICOT AND OAT BLISS BALLS

SERVES
12

PREPARATION
15 MINS

COST PER SERVE
$0.40

320 g dried apricots
½ cup desiccated coconut
1 cup rolled oats
¼ cup coconut oil

NUTRI DETAILS PER SERVE

554 kJ/132 cals	Sat fat: 5.2 g
Protein: 2 g	Carbs: 15.2 g
Fibre: 3 g	Total sugar: 9.4 g
Total fat: 6.5 g	Free sugar: 0 g

Place the apricots in a food processor and blitz until finely chopped.

Set aside 2 tablespoons of the desiccated coconut for rolling the balls.

Add the remaining coconut to the food processor, along with the rolled oats and coconut oil, and blitz until combined.

Shape the mixture into 24 even-sized balls, then roll in the reserved coconut to coat. Two balls is one serve.

Store any leftovers in an airtight container in the fridge for up to 2 weeks or freeze for up to 3 months.

SUITABLE TO FREEZE

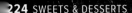

PECAN NUT FUDGE

SERVES	PREPARATION	COOK	COST PER SERVE
20	10 MINS, PLUS COOLING AND CHILLING TIME	5 MINS	$0.31

⅓ cup coconut oil
190 g peanut butter
1 teaspoon liquid stevia
2 teaspoons vanilla extract
salt
½ cup pecans, roughly
  chopped

NUTRI DETAILS PER SERVE

545 kJ/129 cals	Sat fat: 4.4 g
Protein: 3 g	Carbs: 1.1 g
Fibre: 1.4 g	Total sugar: 0.7 g
Total fat: 12.4 g	Free sugar: 0 g

Line a 20 cm x 30 cm slice tin with baking paper.

Place the coconut oil and peanut butter in a saucepan and stir over medium heat for 3 minutes until melted and smooth. Set aside to cool slightly.

When the mixture is cool, stir in the liquid stevia, vanilla and a pinch of salt.

Spread the mixture over the prepared tray and smooth the surface. Sprinkle the pecans over the top and gently press them in.

Refrigerate for 1 hour or until the fudge has set to your desired consistency. Cut into 20 even-sized pieces. One piece is one serve.

Store any leftovers in an airtight container in the fridge for up to 1 week or freeze for up to 2 months.

SUITABLE TO FREEZE

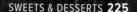

PEANUT BUTTER AND
CHOCOLATE BROWNIE BITES

SERVES
24

PREPARATION
15 MINS, PLUS
SOAKING TIME

COOK
30 MINS, PLUS
COOLING TIME

COST PER SERVE
$0.35

190 g peanut butter
1 cup pitted medjool dates,
    soaked in boiling water for
    10 minutes, then drained
    and pureed
½ cup oat bran
2 free-range eggs
cooking oil spray
60 g dark chocolate
    (70% cocoa solids)
80 g light cream cheese
2 tablespoons reduced-fat
    milk of choice
1 teaspoon vanilla extract
½ cup crushed peanuts

NUTRI DETAILS PER SERVE

609 kJ/145 cals	Sat fat: 2.6 g
Protein: 4.7 g	Carbs: 9 g
Fibre: 1.8 g	Total sugar: 6.4 g
Total fat: 9.8 g	Free sugar: 0 g

Preheat the oven to 180°C and line a 20 cm square slice tin with baking paper.

Place the peanut butter, date puree, oat bran and one egg in a large bowl and mix to form a thick dough.

Press the dough into the base of the prepared tin (the mixture is sticky, so it's a good idea to spray your hands with a little cooking oil first). Bake the peanut butter layer for 12–15 minutes.

Meanwhile, break the chocolate into small pieces and melt in a medium heatproof bowl set over a saucepan of simmering water, stirring occasionally. (Alternatively, melt it in the microwave.) Allow to cool for 3–5 minutes, then stir in the cream cheese, milk, vanilla and remaining egg until smooth.

Remove the peanut butter layer from the oven and pour the chocolate mixture over the top. Sprinkle with the crushed peanuts and bake for a further 10 minutes until a skewer inserted into the centre of the brownie comes out with only a few crumbs clinging to it.

Cool completely in the tin, then cut 24 bite-sized squares. One square is one serve.

Store any leftovers in an airtight container in the fridge for up to 3 days or freeze for up to 1 month.

SUITABLE TO FREEZE

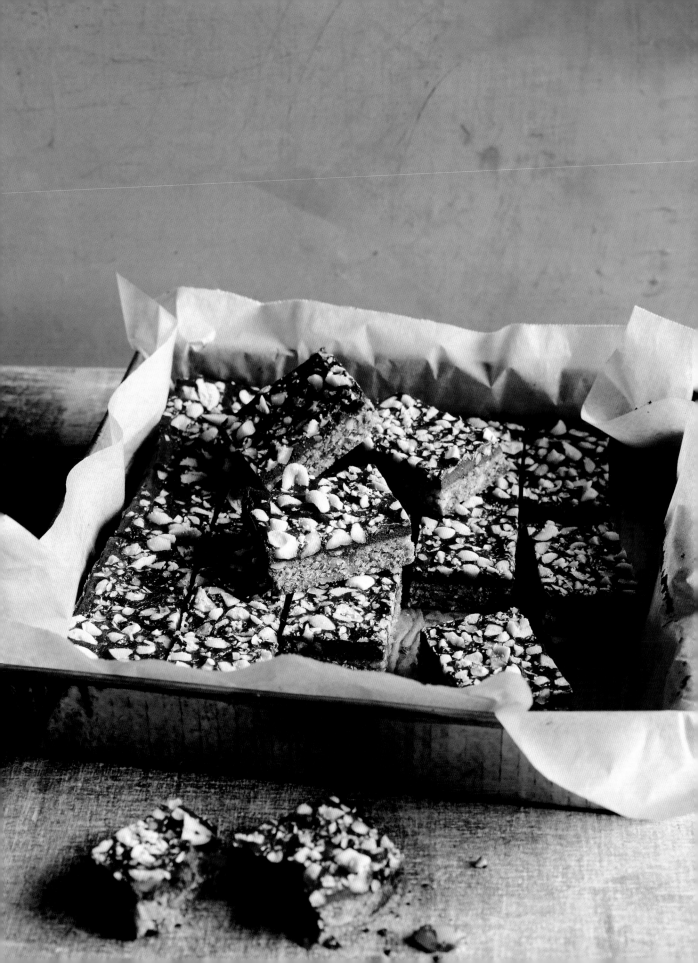

LEMON AND COCONUT SLICE

SERVES
15

PREPARATION
10 MINS, PLUS
FREEZING TIME

COST PER SERVE
$0.90

1 cup almond meal
1 tablespoon finely grated
  lemon zest
⅓ cup lemon juice
2¼ cups desiccated coconut
100 ml coconut oil, melted
1¼ tablespoons honey
300 g coconut yoghurt

NUTRI DETAILS PER SERVE

894 kJ/202 cals	Sat fat: 15.2 g
Protein: 2.4 g	Carbs: 3.9 g
Fibre: 2.2 g	Total sugar: 3.2 g
Total fat: 20.9 g	Free sugar: 1.9 g

Line a standard loaf tin with baking paper.

Place the almond meal, lemon zest and juice, 2 cups of the desiccated coconut, ¼ cup of the melted coconut oil and 1 tablespoon of the honey in a food processor and blitz until well combined. Add a little water if needed to bring the mixture together.

Press the mixture evenly into the prepared tin and place in the freezer for 1 hour until firm.

Place the yoghurt and remaining desiccated coconut, melted coconut oil and honey in the cleaned food processor bowl and blitz until well combined. Pour the mixture over the base layer.

Return the tin to the freezer for another 2 hours until the topping has set.

Cut into 15 even-sized pieces. One piece is one serve.

Store any leftovers in the freezer for up to 2 months. Thaw for about 30 minutes before serving.

SUITABLE TO FREEZE

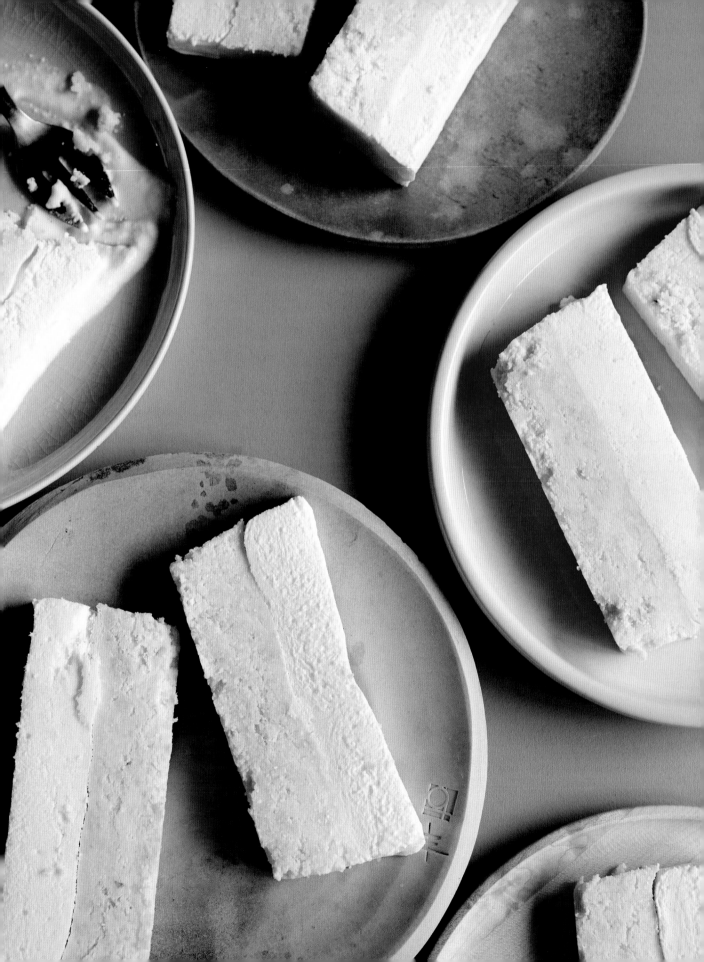

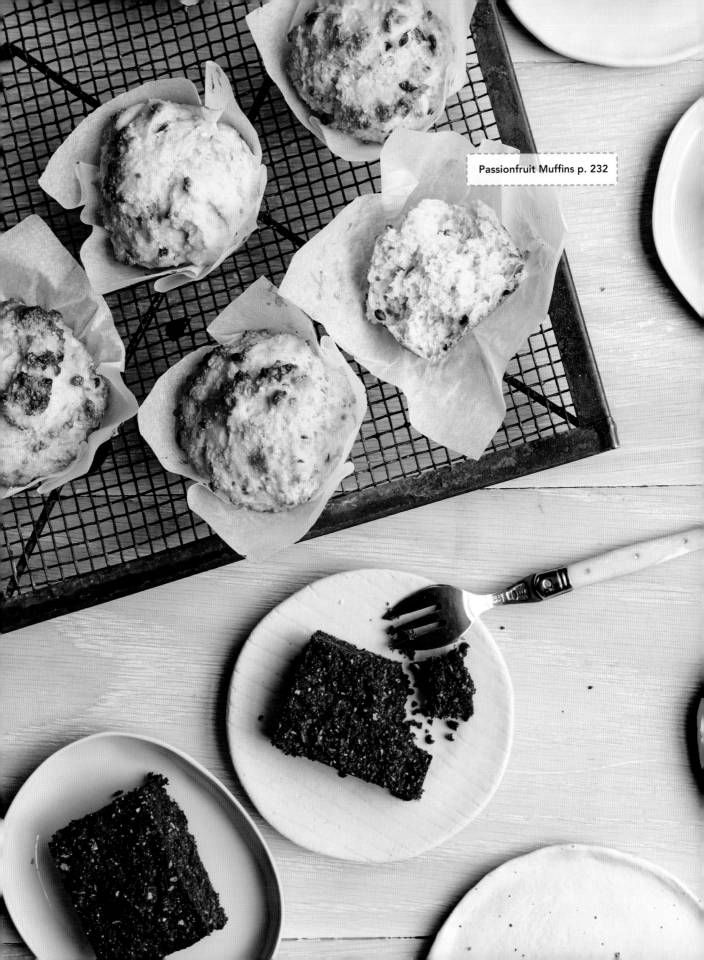

Passionfruit Muffins p. 232

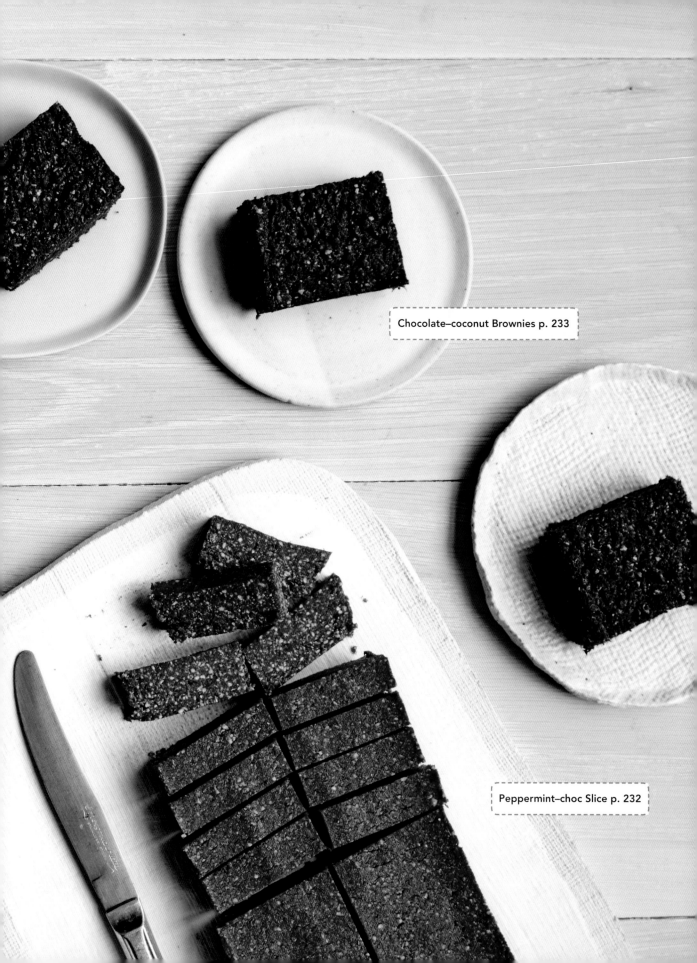

Chocolate–coconut Brownies p. 233

Peppermint–choc Slice p. 232

PASSIONFRUIT MUFFINS

SERVES	PREPARATION	COOK	COST PER SERVE
6	10 MINS	20 MINS	$0.65

½ cup reduced-fat plain Greek yoghurt
1 free-range egg
1 tablespoon honey
2 tablespoons passionfruit pulp
1¼ cups wholemeal self-raising flour
¼ teaspoon baking powder

Preheat the oven to 180°C. Line or lightly grease six holes of a standard muffin tin.

Place the yoghurt, egg, honey, half the passionfruit pulp and ¼ cup of water in a large bowl and whisk to combine. Sift over the flour and baking powder and gently fold through.

Divide the batter evenly among the prepared muffin holes and top with the remaining passionfruit pulp.

Bake for 18–20 minutes until a skewer inserted into the centre of a muffin comes out clean. Cool in the tin for 5 minutes before turning out onto a wire rack to cool completely. One muffin is one serve.

Store any leftover muffins in an airtight container at room temperature for 2–3 days or freeze for up to 2 months.

SUITABLE TO FREEZE

NUTRI DETAILS PER SERVE

554 kJ/132 cals	Sat fat: 0.3 g
Protein: 5.4 g	Carbs: 22.7 g
Fibre: 2.9 g	Total sugar: 5.8 g
Total fat: 1.3 g	Free sugar: 5 g

PEPPERMINT– CHOC SLICE

SERVES	PREPARATION	COST PER SERVE
14	10 MINS, PLUS FREEZING TIME	$0.65

2 cups unsalted cashews
⅓ cup cacao powder
½ cup pitted medjool dates
½ cup desiccated coconut
½ teaspoon peppermint extract
1 tablespoon coconut oil, melted

Line a standard loaf tin with baking paper.

Blitz the cashews to a fine crumb in a food processor. Add the cacao powder and process until well combined.

Add the dates, desiccated coconut, peppermint extract and coconut oil and process to form a sticky dough. Add a splash of water if needed to bring it together.

Spoon the mixture into the prepared tin and press down to smooth the surface.

Freeze for at least 1 hour to firm up. Cut into 28 even-sized pieces. Two pieces is one serve.

Store any leftovers in an airtight container in the fridge for up to 2 weeks or freeze for up to 2 months.

SUITABLE TO FREEZE

NUTRI DETAILS PER SERVE

643 kJ/153 cals	Sat fat: 3.6 g
Protein: 3.6 g	Carbs: 12.5 g
Fibre: 2 g	Total sugar: 5 g
Total fat: 11.3 g	Free sugar: 0 g

CHOCOLATE–COCONUT BROWNIES

SERVES
12

PREPARATION
10 MINS, PLUS
COOLING TIME

COOK
20 MINS

COST PER SERVE
$0.47

150 g dark chocolate
(70% cocoa solids),
broken into pieces
½ cup coconut oil
2 free-range eggs
¾ cup wholemeal self-raising
flour
½ cup coconut sugar
1 teaspoon vanilla extract
2 tablespoons cacao powder
¼ cup desiccated coconut

NUTRI DETAILS PER SERVE

1010 kJ/240 cals	Sat fat: 14 g
Protein: 2.8 g	Carbs: 20.5 g
Fibre: 1.7 g	Total sugar: 15.5 g
Total fat: 17 g	Free sugar: 12 g

Preheat the oven to 200°C and line a 20 cm square cake tin with baking paper.

Place the chocolate and coconut oil in a small saucepan over low heat. Heat slowly, stirring occasionally, for about 5 minutes until melted and smooth. Remove from the heat and allow to cool a little.

Beat the eggs in a large bowl, then stir in the melted chocolate mixture. Add the remaining ingredients and stir until combined.

Spoon the mixture into the prepared tin and bake for 15 minutes until the top is firm. Remove from the oven and allow to cool completely in the tin.

Lift the brownie out of the tin and cut into 12 even-sized pieces. One piece is one serve.

Store any leftovers in an airtight container in the fridge for 4–5 days (the brownies are great reheated in the microwave) or freeze for up to 2 months.

SUITABLE TO FREEZE

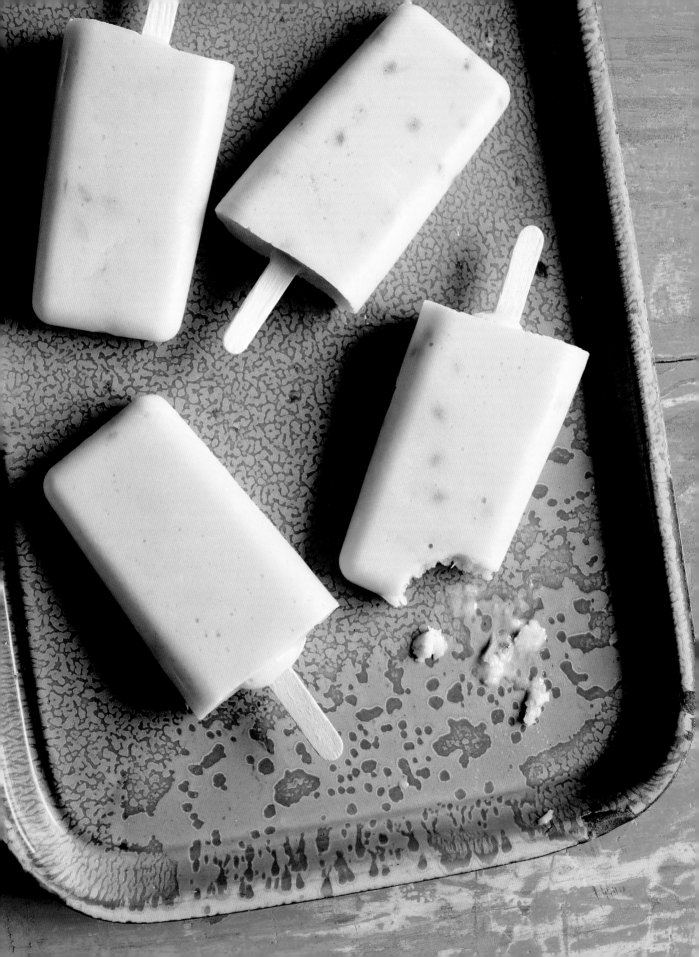

CREAMY PASSIONFRUIT AND MANGO ICE BLOCKS

SERVES
6

PREPARATION
10 MINS, PLUS OVERNIGHT
FREEZING TIME

COST PER SERVE
$1.29

1 cup passionfruit pulp
150 g silken tofu
1 mango (fresh or frozen),
   chopped
1 cup unsweetened
   almond milk
2 tablespoons pure
   maple syrup

NUTRI DETAILS PER SERVE

422 kJ/100 cals	Sat fat: 1 g
Protein: 4 g	Carbs: 13 g
Fibre: 4 g	Total sugar: 12 g
Total fat: 3 g	Free sugar: 5 g

Strain ½ cup of the passionfruit juice, reserving the seeds and remaining juice.

Place all the ingredients, except the reserved passionfruit seeds and juice, in a blender or food processor and blitz until smooth. Stir through the reserved passionfruit seeds and juice.

Pour the mixture into six ice-block moulds and freeze overnight until firm. One ice block is one serve.

Store any leftovers in the freezer for up to 4 months.

SUITABLE TO FREEZE

RASPBERRY AND YOGHURT CAKE

SERVES
8

PREPARATION
20 MINS

COOK
45 MINS

COST PER SERVE
$0.92

2 cups wholemeal self-raising flour
½ teaspoon baking powder
⅓ cup coconut sugar
2 free-range eggs, lightly beaten
½ cup reduced-fat milk of choice
1 cup reduced-fat plain Greek yoghurt
1 teaspoon vanilla extract
½ cup raspberries (fresh or frozen)

ICING

1 cup reduced-fat plain Greek yoghurt
½ cup raspberries (fresh or frozen)
1 tablespoon pure maple syrup

NUTRI DETAILS PER SERVE

884 kJ/211 cals	Sat fat: 2 g
Protein: 8.5 g	Carbs: 37 g
Fibre: 4.7 g	Total sugar: 14.1 g
Total fat: 4.7 g	Free sugar: 10.4 g

Preheat the oven to 180°C. Grease and line a 20 cm round cake tin with baking paper.

Place the flour, baking powder and sugar in a large bowl and whisk to combine. Add the egg, milk, yoghurt and vanilla and stir thoroughly. Fold in the raspberries. (If you are using frozen raspberries, microwave them for 30 seconds to thaw slightly.)

Pour the batter into the prepared tin and bake for 40–45 minutes until firm to touch and a skewer inserted into the centre of the cake comes out clean. Cool in the tin for 5 minutes, then turn out onto a wire rack to cool completely.

To make the icing, start by thickening the yoghurt. Place two clean Chux cloths (or a square of muslin or cheesecloth) on top of 12 sheets of paper towel. Place the yoghurt in the centre, then pull up the sides of the cloth to enclose the yoghurt and twist the top. Wrap the paper towel around the cloth and gently squeeze to remove the excess moisture – the paper towel will become quite damp. Scrape the thickened yoghurt into a small mixing bowl and stir in the raspberries and maple syrup. (If you are using frozen raspberries, microwave them for 30 seconds to thaw slightly.)

Spread the icing over the cooled cake, then cut into eight slices and serve. One slice is one serve.

Store any leftovers in an airtight container in the fridge for 2–3 days or freeze the un-iced cake for up to 2 months.

UN-ICED CAKE IS SUITABLE TO FREEZE

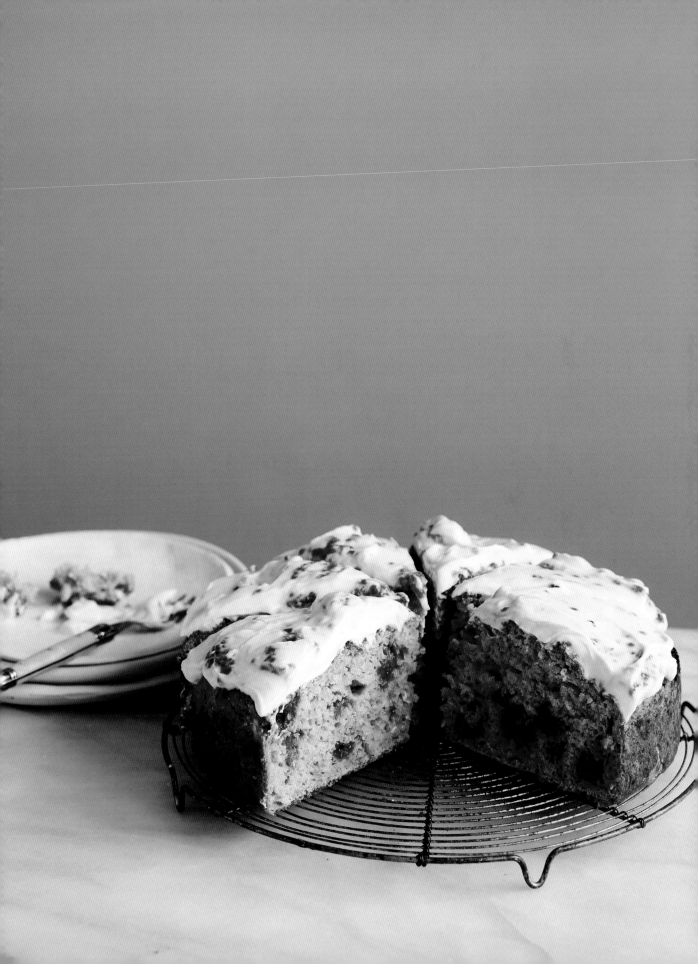

PEAR, CHOCOLATE AND COCONUT CRUMBLE

SERVES
4

PREPARATION
15 MINS

COOK
15 MINS

COST PER SERVE
$0.74

2 pears, peeled, cored
  and diced
2 small bananas, diced
⅓ cup cacao powder
2 ½ tablespoons honey
1 ¼ tablespoons coconut oil
¼ cup wholemeal plain flour
½ cup rolled oats
¼ cup shredded coconut

NUTRI DETAILS PER SERVE

1347 kJ/321 cals	Sat fat: 10.5 g
Protein: 5.2 g	Carbs: 45.4 g
Fibre: 5.3 g	Total sugar: 30 g
Total fat: 12.7 g	Free sugar: 10.3 g

Preheat the oven to 200°C.

Combine the pear, banana, cacao powder, half the honey and
160 ml of water in a small saucepan. Bring to the boil, then reduce
the heat and simmer for 3 minutes to cook the pear. Mash well with
a fork or blend until smooth.

Spoon the chocolate and pear mixture into a round baking dish.

Place the coconut oil and flour in a bowl and rub together to create
coarse crumbs. Mix through the oats and coconut. Sprinkle the
crumble mixture over the chocolate and pear mixture, then drizzle
with the remaining honey.

Bake for 10 minutes until nicely browned on top. Divide evenly
among four bowls and serve.

Store any leftovers in an airtight container in the fridge for 3–4 days
or freeze for up to 2 months.

SUITABLE TO FREEZE

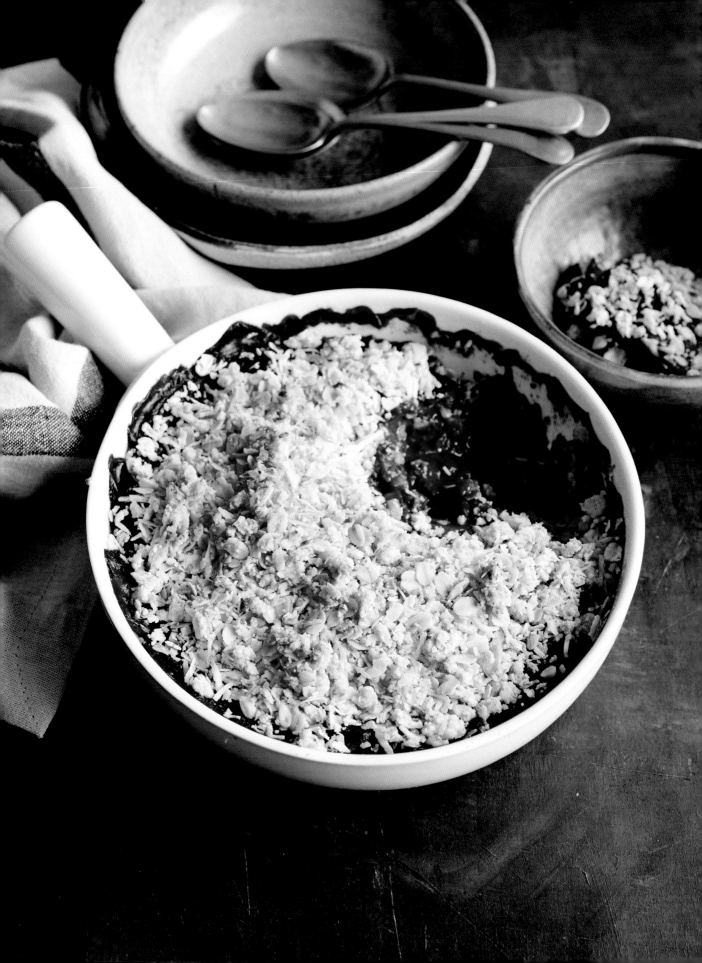

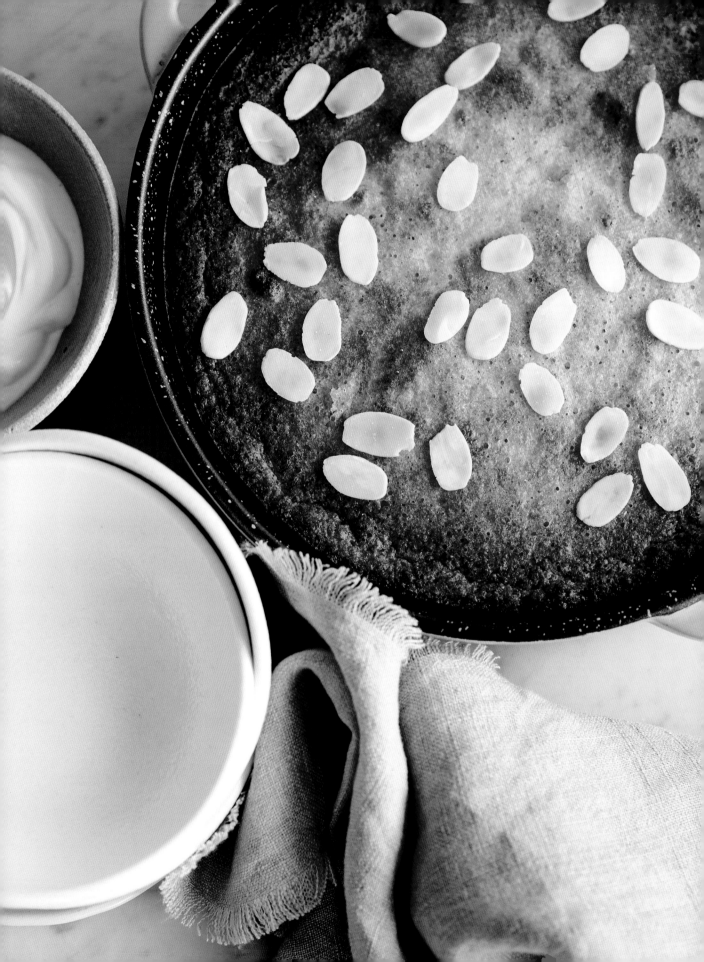

SLOW-COOKED LEMON PUDDING

SERVES
14

PREPARATION
15 MINS

COOK
1 HOUR (4 HOURS IN
A SLOW COOKER)

COST PER SERVE
$0.85

150 g unsalted butter,
   softened, plus extra
   for greasing
1 cup stevia powder
4 free-range eggs
1¼ cups wholemeal self-
   raising flour
1 tablespoon finely grated
   lemon zest
⅓ cup lemon juice
1½ cups unsweetened
   almond milk
2 tablespoons flaked almonds
1 cup reduced-fat plain
   Greek yoghurt

NUTRI DETAILS PER SERVE

669 kJ/159 cals	Sat fat: 6.6 g
Protein: 4.2 g	Carbs: 8.2 g
Fibre: 1.3 g	Total sugar: 1.7 g
Total fat: 11.8 g	Free sugar: 0 g

Beat the butter and stevia until light and fluffy.

Separate one of the eggs and add the yolk to the butter mixture (reserve the egg white for later). Gently mix in one-quarter each of the flour, lemon zest, lemon juice and milk.

Repeat this step three more times until you have added all the egg yolks, flour, lemon zest, lemon juice and milk.

Using clean beaters, beat the egg whites until soft peaks form. Gently fold into the pudding batter.

If cooking in the oven:
Preheat the oven to 180°C and lightly grease a pudding dish. Pour the batter into the dish and bake for 45–60 minutes until golden, moist and cooked through. Scatter over the flaked almonds.

If cooking in a slow cooker:
Lightly grease the slow cooker dish and pour in the batter.
Cover and cook on low for 4 hours until golden, moist and cooked through. Scatter over the flaked almonds.

To serve:
Slice into 14 even-sized pieces. One piece with a dollop of yoghurt is one serve.

Store any leftover pudding in an airtight container in the fridge for 4–5 days or freeze for up to 2 months.

SUITABLE TO FREEZE

CHOC–HAZELNUT FREEZER PIE

SERVES
20

PREPARATION
20 MINS, PLUS
FREEZING TIME

COOK
5 MINS

COST PER SERVE
$0.60

½ cup sunflower seeds
8 dates, pitted
1 cup roasted unsalted
  hazelnuts
2 avocados, mashed
¼ cup pure maple syrup
⅓ cup cacao powder
salt
¼ cup coconut oil
1 teaspoon stevia powder

NUTRI DETAILS PER SERVE

677 kJ/161 cals	Sat fat: 3.6 g
Protein: 2.7 g	Carbs: 6 g
Fibre: 1.9 g	Total sugar: 5.3 g
Total fat: 13.9 g	Free sugar: 2.5 g

Line an 18 cm round springform tin with baking paper.

Place the sunflower seeds, dates and ½ cup of the hazelnuts in a blender and mix until well combined. Press into the base of the prepared tin and place in the freezer to firm up.

In a food processor, blitz ¼ cup of the remaining hazelnuts into a fine meal.

Place the hazelnut meal, avocado, maple syrup, ¼ cup of the cacao powder and a pinch of salt in a blender and mix until smooth. Pour over the base and smooth the surface, then return to the freezer while you make the top layer.

Combine the coconut oil, stevia and remaining cacao powder in a saucepan and stir over low heat until melted and combined. Remove the pie from the freezer and pour over the chocolate layer. Chop the remaining hazelnuts and sprinkle over the top, then return to the freezer for 2 hours.

Cut into 20 slices and serve frozen. One slice is one serve.

Store any leftovers in the freezer for up to 3 months.

SUITABLE TO FREEZE

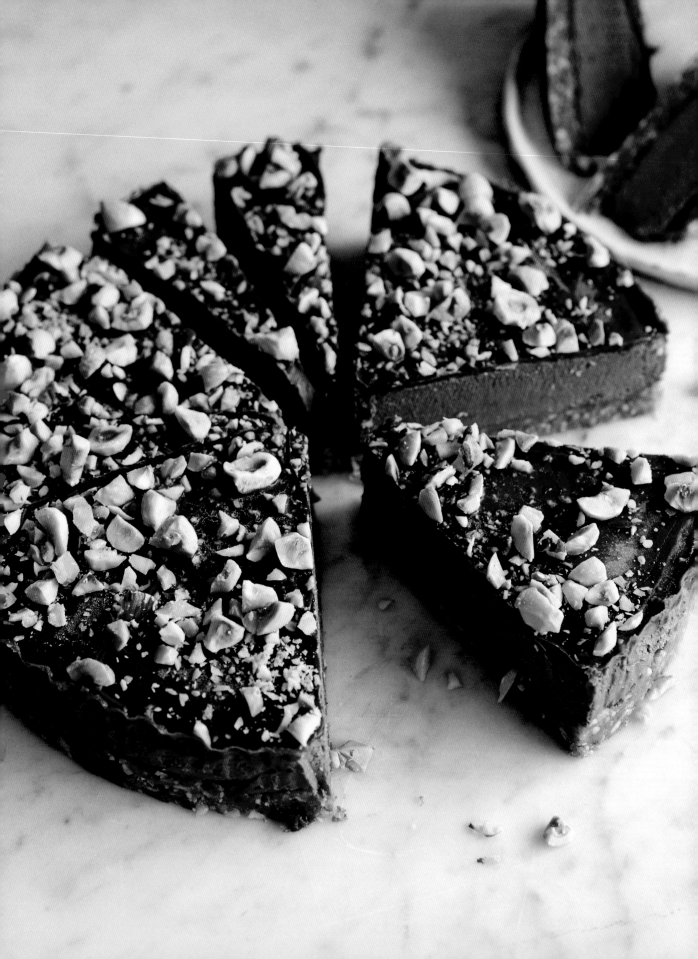

BAKED COFFEE CHEESECAKE

SERVES
10

PREPARATION
20 MINS

COOK
30 MINS, PLUS COOLING
AND CHILLING TIME

COST PER SERVE
$0.51

¼ cup unsalted macadamias
¼ cup almonds
¼ cup desiccated coconut
1 tablespoon coconut oil
250 g light cream cheese,
    at room temperature
½ teaspoon instant coffee
    granules
1½ tablespoons coconut
    cream
1 free-range egg
¼ cup stevia powder
1 teaspoon vanilla extract

NUTRI DETAILS PER SERVE

581 kJ/138 cals	Sat fat: 5.1 g
Protein: 3.8 g	Carbs: 1.5 g
Fibre: 0.9 g	Total sugar: 1.5 g
Total fat: 13 g	Free sugar: 0 g

Preheat the oven to 160°C and line a 20 cm springform cake tin with baking paper.

Place the macadamias and almonds in a food processor and blitz to form a fine meal.

Add the desiccated coconut and coconut oil and blitz again on medium speed to combine.

Transfer the mixture to the prepared tin and press down evenly using the back of a metal spoon. Bake for 8–10 minutes until just starting to brown. Remove from the oven and set aside to cool.

Increase the oven temperature to 175°C.

Place the cream cheese, coffee, coconut cream, egg, stevia and vanilla in the cleaned food processor bowl and blend until smooth. Pour the filling over the cooled base and smooth the surface.

Bake for 20 minutes until the cream filling is a little wobbly in the centre. Allow to cool, then cover and place in the fridge for at least 2 hours until firm and set.

Slice into 10 even-sized pieces. One piece is one serve.

Store any leftovers in an airtight container in the fridge for 3–4 days or freeze for up to 2 months.

SUITABLE TO FREEZE

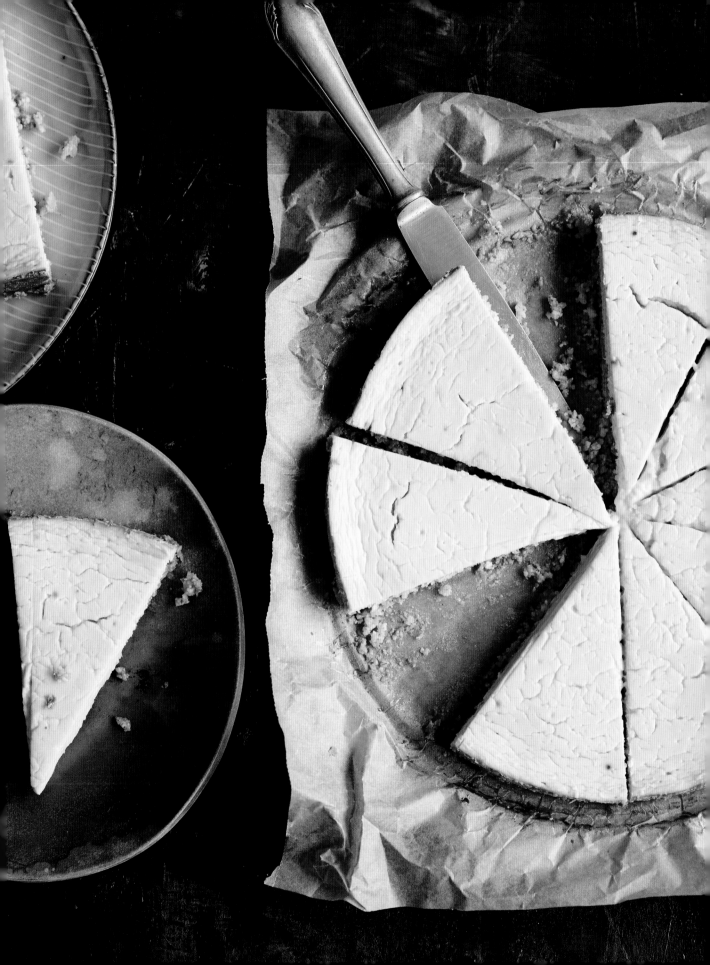

CONVERSION CHARTS

Measuring cups and spoons may vary slightly from one country to another, but the difference is generally not enough to affect a recipe. All cup and spoon measures are level.

One Australian metric measuring cup holds 250 ml (8 fl oz), one Australian tablespoon holds 20 ml (4 teaspoons) and one Australian metric teaspoon holds 5 ml. North America, New Zealand and the UK use a 15 ml (3-teaspoon) tablespoon.

LENGTH

METRIC	IMPERIAL
3 mm	⅛ inch
6 mm	¼ inch
1 cm	½ inch
2.5 cm	1 inch
5 cm	2 inches
18 cm	7 inches
20 cm	8 inches
23 cm	9 inches
25 cm	10 inches
30 cm	12 inches

LIQUID MEASURES

ONE AMERICAN PINT	ONE IMPERIAL PINT
500 ml (16 fl oz)	600 ml (20 fl oz)

CUP	METRIC	IMPERIAL
⅛ cup	30 ml	1 fl oz
¼ cup	60 ml	2 fl oz
⅓ cup	80 ml	2½ fl oz
½ cup	125 ml	4 fl oz
⅔ cup	160 ml	5 fl oz
¾ cup	180 ml	6 fl oz
1 cup	250 ml	8 fl oz
2 cups	500 ml	16 fl oz
2¼ cups	560 ml	20 fl oz
4 cups	1 litre	32 fl oz

DRY MEASURES

The most accurate way to measure dry ingredients is to weigh them. However, if using a cup, add the ingredient loosely to the cup and level with a knife; don't compact the ingredient unless the recipe requests 'firmly packed'.

METRIC	IMPERIAL
15 g	½ oz
30 g	1 oz
60 g	2 oz
125 g	4 oz (¼ lb)
185 g	6 oz
250 g	8 oz (½ lb)
375 g	12 oz (¾ lb)
500 g	16 oz (1 lb)
1 kg	32 oz (2 lb)

OVEN TEMPERATURES

CELSIUS	FAHRENHEIT
100°C	200°F
120°C	250°F
150°C	300°F
160°C	325°F
180°C	350°F
200°C	400°F
220°C	425°F

CELSIUS	GAS MARK
110°C	¼
130°C	½
140°C	1
150°C	2
170°C	3
180°C	4
190°C	5
200°C	6
220°C	7
230°C	8
240°C	9
250°C	10

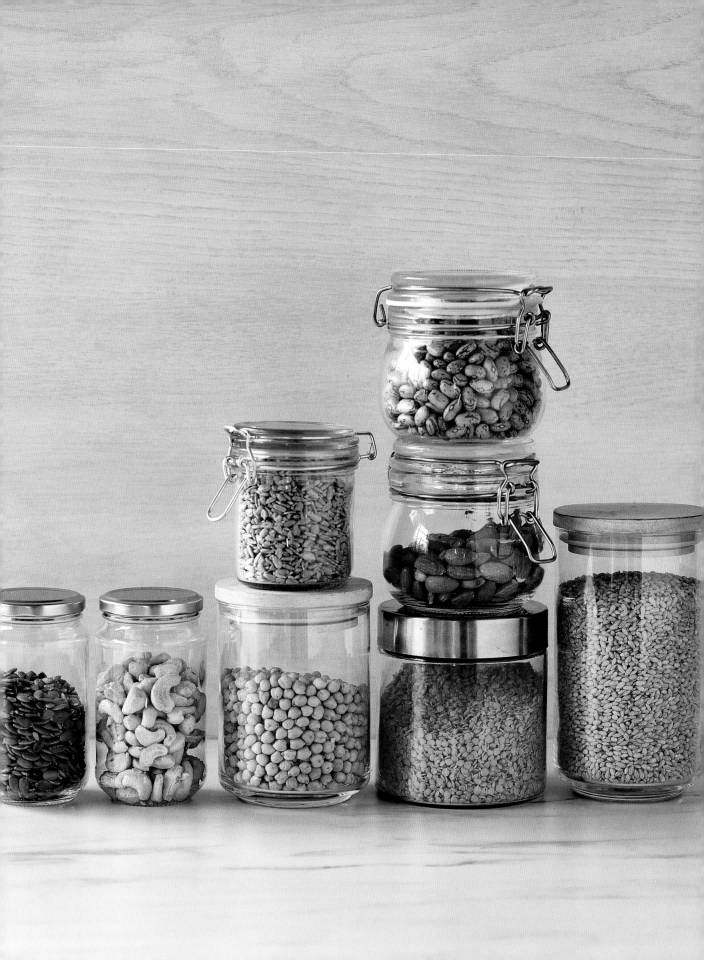

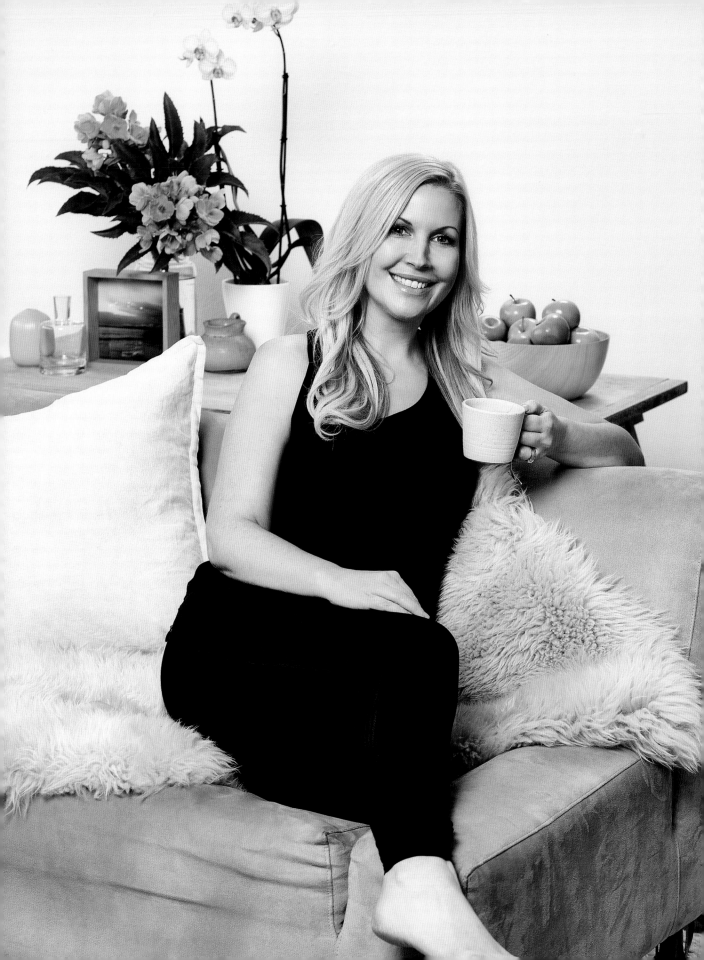

THANKS

Without the help of the following amazing people, none of this would have been possible:

The fabulous team at Plum and Pan Macmillan, especially Mary Small, Clare Marshall and Rachel Carter, all of your guidance and expertise in bringing this book to life is truly inspiring.

The wonderful creative team: photographers Steve Brown and Chris Middleton, designer Kirby Armstrong, stylists Vanessa Austin and Lee Blaylock. Turning my vision into a beautiful reality is so humbling.

The talented home economics team: Sarah Mayoh, Caroline Griffiths and Rachael Lane, without you the stunning images in this book wouldn't be as beautiful as they truly are.

My team of nutritionists, including Cheree Sheldon, Nikki Boswell, Elisha Danine, Shirley De Jesus, Sarina Darenzo: thank you all for creating some of the most delicious and healthy meals for our busy mums.

To The Healthy Mummy team, I couldn't have done this without all of your hard work day in and day out. A special thanks to Isabella Jolly, Georga Holdich and Rachael Javes for being such a huge part of creating this amazing book.

Marlene Richardson, thank you for working so closely with me on the book.

Of course, thank you to The Healthy Mummy community of hundreds of thousands of busy mums; you are my motivation and without you The Healthy Mummy wouldn't be what it is today.

And last, but definitely not least, to my my husband, John, and my two boys, Kai and Jake – thank you for always supporting me and being such a huge part of my Healthy Mummy journey. I couldn't do what I do without you!

Rhian

Founder, The Healthy Mummy
healthymummy.com

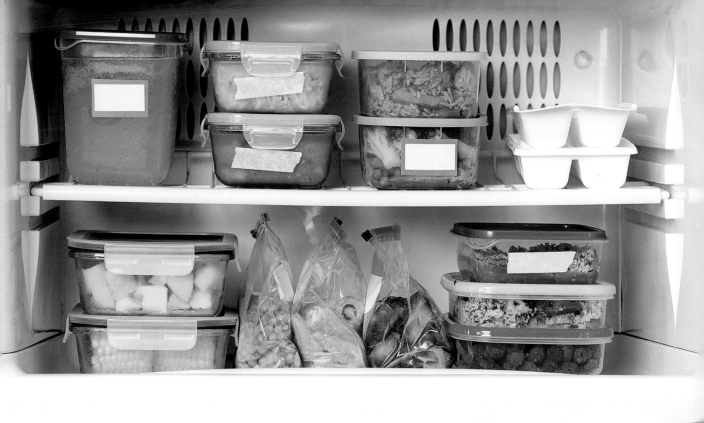
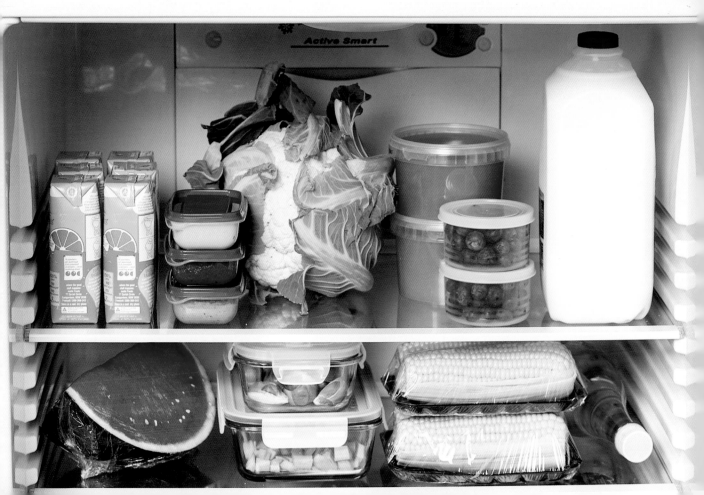

INDEX

A

Apple and blueberry cornbread 46
apples
    Apple and blueberry cornbread 46
    Fruity breakfast slice 61
    Tropical green smoothie 86
Apricot and oat bliss balls 224
Asian pork and veggie rice balls 216
asparagus
    Asparagus and chicken mini
        quiches 213
    Buddha bowl 107
Asparagus and chicken mini quiches 213
avocados
    Chicken and jalapeno poppers with
        guacamole 182
    Choc–hazelnut freezer pie 242
    Mexican breakfast wrap 74
    Mexican quinoa, chickpea and corn
        casserole 150

B

bacon
    Bacon and egg with veggie hash 67
    Bacon and zucchini muffins 72
    Bacon pasta salad 117
    Gourmet scrambled eggs 66
    Turmeric egg and bacon wrap 79
Bacon and egg with veggie hash 67
Bacon and zucchini muffins 72
Bacon pasta salad 117
Baked cheese and tomato risotto 140
Baked coffee cheesecake 244
Baked oats with banana and berries 51
Baked sweet potatoes with spinach
    and feta 176
bakes
    Baked oats with banana and berries 51
    Breakfast tray bake 62
    Cheesy veggie bake 180
    Sausage and vegetable pasta bake 136
    Zucchini and ricotta bake 64
bananas 21
    Baked oats with banana and berries 51
    Bright eyes smoothie 86
    Choc–banana breakfast bowl 48
    Coco–banana bliss smoothie 95
    Coconut rough smoothie 90
    Fruity breakfast slice 61
    Gingerbread pancakes 54
    Minty coconut smoothie 87
    Mocha banana bread 57
    Oven-baked maple and banana
        French toast 46
    Pear, chocolate and coconut
        crumble 238
    Raspberry–oat smoothie 94
Basal Metabolic Rate (BMR) 8, 9
beans
    Chicken burrito bowls 167
    Mexican breakfast wrap 74
    Slow-cooked beef nachos 200

Slow-cooked vegetable and
    tortellini soup 126
    see also green beans
beef 21
    Beef chow mein 166
    Beef stroganoff with polenta 168
    Beef, lentil and veggie soup 130
    Hidden veg bolognese 40
    Hidden veg bolognese pie 196
    Hidden veg bolognese potatoes 197
    Open burger with the lot 164
    Slow-cooked beef nachos 200
    Zoodles with hidden veg bolognese 144
Beef chow mein 166
Beef stroganoff with polenta 168
Beef, lentil and veggie soup 130
beetroot
    Beetroot, mint and cashew dip 207
    Open burger with the lot 164
Beetroot, mint and cashew dip 207
berries 22
    Baked oats with banana and berries 51
    Silky skin smoothie 95
    see also blueberries, raspberries,
        strawberries
bliss balls, Apricot and oat 224
blueberries
    Apple and blueberry cornbread 46
    Bright eyes smoothie 86
    Fruit fusion smoothie 90
    Fruity breakfast slice 61
    Peanut butter granola 52
bolognese, Hidden veg 40
bolognese, Zoodles with hidden veg 144
bowls
    Buddha bowl 107
    Cajun chicken salad bowl 114
    Chia, mango and pistachio breakfast
        bowl 49
    Chicken burrito bowls 167
    Choc–banana breakfast bowl 48
    Spiced chickpea bowl 108
bread
    Apple and blueberry cornbread 46
    Cheese and olive pinwheels 210
    Mocha banana bread 57
Breakfast tray bake 62
Bright eyes smoothie 86
broccoli
    Cheesy veggie bake 180
    Refreshing detox salad 104
    Spiced chickpea bowl 108
    Spicy broccoli and cheese pikelets 208
brownie bites, Peanut butter and
    chocolate 226
brownies, Chocolate–coconut 233
brussels sprouts
    Roasted rainbow veggie breakfast
        salad 80
    Roasted rainbow veggie, kale and
        quinoa salad 100
    Roasted rainbow veggies 37
    Spiced chicken and roasted rainbow
        veggie tacos 191

Buddha bowl 107
budget shopping 8, 12, 18
budget, household 32–33
bulk cooking 8, 10, 12, 26
bulk shopping 8, 10, 18–21, 30
bulk storing 30
burger, Open, with the lot 164

C

cabbage
    Bacon pasta salad 117
    Beef chow mein 166
    Fish tacos with coleslaw 179
    Hidden veg bolognese potatoes 197
    Open burger with the lot 164
    Refreshing detox salad 104
Cajun chicken 39
Cajun chicken meatballs 215
Cajun chicken pizzas 189
Cajun chicken salad bowl 114
cakes
    Baked coffee cheesecake 244
    Raspberry and yoghurt cake 236
calories 8
canned foods 21
capsicums
    Bacon and egg with veggie hash 67
    Bacon pasta salad 117
    Chicken burrito bowls 167
    Greek pizza muffin 70
    Greek tuna salad 116
    Hidden veg bolognese 40
    Hidden veg bolognese pie 196
    Hidden veg bolognese potatoes 197
    Mexican quinoa, chickpea and corn
        casserole 150
    Ratatouille lasagne 135
    Roasted rainbow veggie breakfast
        salad 80
    Roasted rainbow veggie, kale and
        quinoa salad 100
    Roasted rainbow veggies 37
    Simple roasted veggie salad 105
    Slow-cooked beef nachos 200
    Spiced chicken and roasted rainbow
        veggie tacos 191
    Zoodles with hidden veg
        bolognese 144
carrots
    Asian pork and veggie rice balls 216
    Bacon pasta salad 117
    Beef chow mein 166
    Beef, lentil and veggie soup 130
    Beetroot, mint and cashew dip 207
    Cajun chicken meatballs 215
    Cheesy chicken meatballs in tomato
        and spinach sauce 156
    Cheesy veggie bake 180
    Coconutty pumpkin soup 128
    Creamy spring onion dip 206
    Fish tacos with coleslaw 179
    Hot and spicy hummus 206
    Lamb and lentil curry 41

Lamb and lentil curry pasties 199
Lamb and lentil curry with coriander rice 171
Lamb and lentil curry-stuffed zucchini 194
Lentil shepherd's pie 174
Pork pad Thai 146
Pulled pork, rice and kale salad 111
Refreshing detox salad 104
Sausage and vegetable pasta bake 136
Slow-cooked vegetable and tortellini soup 126
Sweet chilli tuna rice paper rolls 123
Thai chicken meatloaf 184
Veggie-loaded fritters 69
case studies 34–35
casserole, Mexican quinoa, chickpea and corn 150

cauliflower
Cheesy veggie bake 180
Refreshing detox salad 104

celery
Asian pork and veggie rice balls 216
Coconutty pumpkin soup 128
Hidden veg bolognese 40
Hidden veg bolognese pie 196
Hidden veg bolognese potatoes 197
Slow-cooked vegetable and tortellini soup 126
Zoodles with hidden veg bolognese 144

cheese
Bacon and zucchini muffins 72
Baked cheese and tomato risotto 140
Baked coffee cheesecake 244
Baked sweet potatoes with spinach and feta 176
Cajun chicken meatballs 215
Cajun chicken pizzas 189
Cheese and olive pinwheels 210
Cheesy chicken meatballs in tomato and spinach sauce 156
Cheesy veggie bake 180
Chicken and corn fritters 154
Chicken and jalapeno poppers with guacamole 182
Corn and ham breakfast slice 77
Creamy spring onion dip 206
Greek pizza muffin 70
Ham, spinach and feta pizzas 189
Hawaiian melts 78
Hidden veg bolognese potatoes 197
Lemon–raspberry muffins 60
Lentil shepherd's pie 174
Mini cheese, ham and quinoa muffins 212
Mushroom and sun-dried tomato mini frittatas 73
Open burger with the lot 164
Peanut butter and chocolate brownie bites 226
Potato salad with spinach and chorizo 112
Pumpkin and feta tart 188
Ratatouille lasagne 135
Sausage and vegetable pasta bake 136
Simple roasted veggie salad 105
Slow-cooked beef nachos 200

Slow-cooked vegetable and tortellini soup 126
Spicy broccoli and cheese pikelets 208
Super-quick ham, cheese and tomato quiche 122
Tuna and pumpkin mac and cheese 141
Veggie-loaded fritters 69
Zucchini and ricotta bake 64
Cheese and olive pinwheels 210
Cheesy chicken meatballs in tomato and spinach sauce 156
Cheesy veggie bake 180
cherries: Porridge with vanilla–cherry compote 60
Chia, mango and pistachio breakfast bowl 49
chicken 21, 22
Asparagus and chicken mini quiches 213
Cajun chicken 39
Cajun chicken meatballs 215
Cajun chicken pizzas 189
Cajun chicken salad bowl 114
Cheesy chicken meatballs in tomato and spinach sauce 156
Chicken and corn fritters 154
Chicken and jalapeno poppers with guacamole 182
Chicken burrito bowls 167
Chicken caesar wrap 119
Chicken tikka with rice 160
Mediterranean chicken and vegetable pasta 138
Roasted dijon chicken 181
Spiced chicken and roasted rainbow veggie tacos 191
Spicy chicken and corn soup 129
Thai chicken meatloaf 184
Chicken and corn fritters 154
Chicken and jalapeno poppers with guacamole 182
Chicken burrito bowls 167
Chicken caesar wrap 119
Chicken tikka with rice 160
chickpeas
Buddha bowl 107
Hot and spicy hummus 206
Mexican quinoa, chickpea and corn casserole 150
Spiced chickpea bowl 108
Sweet potato and chickpea curry 160
Choc–hazelnut freezer pie 242
Choc–marshmallow slice 220
Choc–banana breakfast bowl 48
chocolate
Choc–banana breakfast bowl 48
Choc–hazelnut freezer pie 242
Choc–marshmallow slice 220
Chocolate–coconut brownies 233
Chocolate–raspberry smoothie 87
Coconut rough smoothie 90
Mocha banana bread 57
Peanut butter and chocolate brownie bites 226
Pear, chocolate and coconut crumble 238
Peppermint–choc slice 232

Chocolate–coconut brownies 233
Chocolate–raspberry smoothie 87
chow mein, Beef 166
Coco–banana bliss smoothie 95
coconut
Apricot and oat bliss balls 224
Baked coffee cheesecake 244
Choc–marshmallow slice 220
Chocolate–coconut brownies 233
Coco–banana bliss smoothie 95
Coconut rough smoothie 90
Coconut–date loaf 222
Lemon and coconut slice 228
Mango, coconut and chilli prawns 153
Minty coconut smoothie 87
Pear, chocolate and coconut crumble 238
Peppermint–choc slice 232
Coconut rough smoothie 90
Coconut–date loaf 222
Coconutty pumpkin soup 128
conversion charts 246
cooking in bulk 8, 10, 12, 26
corn
Beef, lentil and veggie soup 130
Chicken and corn fritters 154
Chicken burrito bowls 167
Corn and ham breakfast slice 77
Mexican quinoa, chickpea and corn casserole 150
Spicy chicken and corn soup 129
Corn and ham breakfast slice 77
cornbread, Apple and blueberry 46
Creamy passionfruit and mango ice blocks 235
Creamy spring onion dip 206
crumble, Pear, chocolate and coconut 238
cucumber
Chicken and corn fritters 154
Flash-fried squid with rocket and pineapple 152
Greek tuna salad 116
Hot and spicy hummus 206
Tropical green smoothie 86
Turkey and salad sub 123
Zesty Greek salad with pulled pork 110
curries
Lamb and lentil curry 41
Lamb and lentil curry with coriander rice 171
Slow-cooked fish curry with pappadums 161
Sweet potato and chickpea curry 160

D
dates
Choc–hazelnut freezer pie 242
Choc–marshmallow slice 220
Coconut–date loaf 222
Peanut butter and chocolate brownie bites 226
Peppermint–choc slice 232
dips
Beetroot, mint and cashew dip 207
Creamy spring onion dip 206
Hot and spicy hummus 206
Sweet potato fries with garlicky dip 207

E

eating out 32
eggplant
    Mediterranean chicken and vegetable
        pasta 138
    Ratatouille lasagne 135
eggs 21
    Asparagus and chicken mini quiches 213
    Bacon and egg with veggie hash 67
    Chicken caesar wrap 119
    Corn and ham breakfast slice 77
    Gourmet scrambled eggs 66
    Mushroom and sun-dried tomato mini
        frittatas 73
    Open burger with the lot 164
    Pork pad Thai 146
    Potato salad with spinach and
        chorizo 112
    Pumpkin and feta tart 188
    Roasted rainbow veggie breakfast
        salad 80
    Spicy chicken and corn soup 129
    Super-quick ham, cheese and tomato
        quiche 122
    Thai chicken meatloaf 184
    Turmeric egg and bacon wrap 79
Energising smoothie 96
exercise 8, 32

F

fish 21
    Fish tacos with coleslaw 179
    Slow-cooked fish curry with
        pappadums 161
    see also tuna
Fish tacos with coleslaw 179
Flash-fried squid with rocket and
    pineapple 152
French toast, Oven-baked maple and
    banana 46
frittatas, Mushroom and sun-dried
    tomato mini 73
fritters, Chicken and corn 154
fritters, Veggie-loaded 69
frozen foods 22
Fruit fusion smoothie 90
Fruity breakfast slice 61
fudge, Pecan nut 225

G

Gingerbread pancakes 54
Gourmet scrambled eggs 66
granola, Peanut butter 52
Greek pizza muffin 70
Greek tuna salad 116
green beans
    Beef chow mein 166
    Beef stroganoff with polenta 168
    Hoisin pork with greens and rice 193
    Lamb and lentil curry 41
    Lamb and lentil curry pasties 199
    Lamb and lentil curry with coriander
        rice 171
    Lamb and lentil curry-stuffed
        zucchini 194
    Roasted dijon chicken 181

Slow-cooked fish curry with
    pappadums 161
Slow-cooked vegetable and
    tortellini soup 126

H

Ham, spinach and feta pizzas 189
Hawaiian melts 78
Healthy Mummy, The 7, 8, 34–35
Hidden veg bolognese 40
Hidden veg bolognese pie 196
Hidden veg bolognese potatoes 197
Hoisin pork with greens and rice 193
Hot and spicy hummus 206
household budget 32–33

I

icing 236
Immunity-boosting smoothie 91
ingredient swaps 12, 18, 22
ingredients, staple 21

K

kale
    Cajun chicken salad bowl 114
    Pulled pork, rice and kale salad 111
    Roasted rainbow veggie, kale and
        quinoa salad 100
    Spiced chickpea bowl 108
    Sweet potato and chickpea curry 160
kiwi fruit: Fruit fusion smoothie 90

L

lamb
    Lamb and lentil curry 41
    Lamb and lentil curry pasties 199
    Lamb and lentil curry with coriander
        rice 171
    Lamb and lentil curry-stuffed
        zucchini 194
lasagne, Ratatouille 135
Lemon and coconut slice 228
Lemon–raspberry muffins 60
Lentil shepherd's pie 174
lentils 22
    Beef, lentil and veggie soup 130
    Lamb and lentil curry 41
    Lamb and lentil curry pasties 199
    Lamb and lentil curry with coriander
        rice 171
    Lamb and lentil curry-stuffed
        zucchini 194
    Lentil shepherd's pie 174
loaf, Coconut–date 220
lunchboxes 33

M

mango
    Chia, mango and pistachio breakfast
        bowl 49
    Creamy passionfruit and mango ice
        blocks 235
    Mango–passionfruit smoothie 97
    Mango, coconut and chilli prawns 153
Mango–passionfruit smoothie 97

Mango, coconut and chilli prawns 153
meal planning 10–12, 18
    sample 7-day meal plan 14–15
    sample 7-day meal plan shopping
        list 16
meal prep 18, 26
meal prep tools 28–29
meat, cheaper cuts 12, 21
meatballs
    Cajun chicken meatballs 215
    Cheesy chicken meatballs in tomato
        and spinach sauce 156
    Turkey meatballs and spaghetti 143
meatloaf, Thai chicken 184
Mediterranean chicken and vegetable
    pasta 138
Mexican breakfast wrap 74
Mexican quinoa, chickpea and corn
    casserole 150
milk, UHT 21
Mini cheese, ham and quinoa muffins 212
Minty coconut smoothie 87
Mocha banana bread 57
muffins
    Bacon and zucchini muffin 72
    Greek pizza muffin 70
    Lemon–raspberry muffins 60
    Mini cheese, ham and quinoa
        muffins 212
    Passionfruit muffins 232
Mushroom and sun-dried tomato mini
    frittatas 73
mushrooms
    Beef stroganoff with polenta 168
    Breakfast tray bake 62
    Chicken burrito bowls 167
    Mushroom and sun-dried tomato
        mini frittatas 73

N

nachos, Slow-cooked beef 200
nectarines: Fruit fusion smoothie 90
nuts
    Baked coffee cheesecake 244
    Beetroot, mint and cashew dip 207
    Chia, mango and pistachio breakfast
        bowl 49
    Choc–banana breakfast bowl 48
    Choc–hazelnut freezer pie 242
    Energising smoothie 96
    Peanut butter and chocolate brownie
        bites 226
    Peanut butter granola 52
    Pecan nut fudge 225
    Peppermint–choc slice 232
    Refreshing detox salad 104
    Slow-cooked lemon pudding 241
    Tuna, roasted pumpkin and brown
        rice salad 102

O

oats, Baked, with banana and berries 51
olives
    Cheese and olive pinwheels 210
    Greek pizza muffin 70
    Greek tuna salad 116
Open burger with the lot 164

oranges: Recovery smoothie 94
Oven-baked maple and banana
    French toast 46

P

pad Thai, Pork 146
pancakes, Gingerbread 54
pantry staples 24–25
parsnips
    Roasted rainbow veggie breakfast
        salad 80
    Roasted rainbow veggie, kale and
        quinoa salad 100
    Roasted rainbow veggies 37
    Spiced chicken and roasted rainbow
        veggie tacos 191
passionfruit
    Creamy passionfruit and mango ice
        blocks 235
    Mango–passionfruit smoothie 97
    Passionfruit muffins 232
Passionfruit muffins 232
pasta 21
    Bacon pasta salad 117
    Mediterranean chicken and vegetable
        pasta 138
    Ratatouille lasagne 135
    Sausage and vegetable pasta bake 136
    Slow-cooked vegetable and tortellini
        soup 126
    Tuna and pumpkin mac and cheese 141
    Turkey meatballs and spaghetti 143
pasties, Lamb and lentil curry 199
peas
    Beef, lentil and veggie soup 130
    Cheesy chicken meatballs in tomato
        and spinach sauce 156
    Lentil shepherd's pie 174
    Slow-cooked fish curry with
        pappadums 161
Peaches and cream smoothie 97
Peanut butter and chocolate brownie
    bites 226
Peanut butter and jelly smoothie 91
Peanut butter granola 52
Pear, chocolate and coconut crumble 238
Pecan nut fudge 225
Peppermint–choc slice 232
pies
    Lentil shepherd's pie 174
    Choc–hazelnut freezer pie 242
    Hidden veg bolognese pie 196
pikelets, Spicy broccoli and cheese 208
pineapple
    Flash-fried squid with rocket and
        pineapple 152
    Hawaiian melts 78
    Tropical green smoothie 86
pizzas
    Cajun chicken pizzas 189
    Greek pizza muffin 70
    Ham, spinach and feta pizzas 189
pork
    Asian pork and veggie rice balls 216
    Chicken caesar wrap 119
    Corn and ham breakfast slice 77
    Ham, spinach and feta pizzas 189
    Hawaiian melts 78
    Hidden veg bolognese 40

Hidden veg bolognese pie 196
Hidden veg bolognese potatoes 197
Hoisin pork with greens and rice 193
Mini cheese, ham and quinoa
    muffins 212
Pork pad Thai 146
Pulled pork 38
Pulled pork and spinach sloppy
    joes 163
Pulled pork, rice and kale salad 111
Super-quick ham, cheese and tomato
    quiche 122
Zesty Greek salad with pulled pork 110
Zoodles with hidden veg bolognese 144
Pork pad Thai 146
Porridge with vanilla–cherry compote 60
porridge, Salted caramel 61
Potato salad with spinach and chorizo 112
potatoes
    Beef, lentil and veggie soup 130
    Hidden veg bolognese potatoes 197
    Lamb and lentil curry 41
    Lamb and lentil curry pasties 199
    Lamb and lentil curry with coriander
        rice 171
    Lamb and lentil curry-stuffed
        zucchini 194
    Potato salad with spinach and
        chorizo 112
prawns: Mango, coconut and chilli
    prawns 153
pudding, Slow-cooked lemon 241
Pulled pork 38
Pulled pork and spinach sloppy joes 163
Pulled pork, rice and kale salad 111
pumpkin
    Buddha bowl 107
    Coconutty pumpkin soup 128
    Hidden veg bolognese 40
    Hidden veg bolognese pie 196
    Hidden veg bolognese potatoes 197
    Pumpkin and feta tart 188
    Roasted rainbow veggie breakfast
        salad 80
    Roasted rainbow veggie, kale and
        quinoa salad 100
    Roasted rainbow veggies 37
    Sausage and vegetable pasta bake 136
    Simple roasted veggie salad 105
    Slow-cooked vegetable and tortellini
        soup 126
    Spiced chicken and roasted rainbow
        veggie tacos 191
    Tuna and pumpkin mac and cheese 141
    Tuna, roasted pumpkin and brown rice
        salad 102
    Zoodles with hidden veg bolognese 144
Pumpkin and feta tart 188

Q

quiche, Super-quick ham, cheese and
    tomato 122
quiches, Asparagus and chicken mini 213
quinoa
    Buddha bowl 107
    Cajun chicken salad bowl 114
    Mexican quinoa, chickpea and corn
        casserole 150

Mini cheese, ham and quinoa
    muffins 212
Roasted rainbow veggie, kale and
    quinoa salad 100

R

raspberries
    Chocolate–raspberry smoothie 87
    icing 236
    Lemon–raspberry muffins 60
    Raspberry and yoghurt cake 236
    Raspberry–oat smoothie 94
Raspberry and yoghurt cake 236
Raspberry–oat smoothie 94
Ratatouille lasagne 135
Recovery smoothie 94
Refreshing detox salad 104
rice 21
    Asian pork and veggie rice balls 216
    Baked cheese and tomato risotto 140
    Chicken burrito bowls 167
    Chicken tikka with rice 160
    Hoisin pork with greens and rice 193
    Lamb and lentil curry with coriander
        rice 171
    Pulled pork, rice and kale salad 111
    Sweet potato and chickpea curry 160
    Tuna, roasted pumpkin and brown rice
        salad 102
rice paper rolls, Sweet chilli tuna 123
risotto, Baked cheese and tomato 140
Roasted dijon chicken 181
Roasted rainbow veggie breakfast salad 80
Roasted rainbow veggie, kale and quinoa
    salad 100
Roasted rainbow veggies 37

S

salads
    Bacon pasta salad 117
    Cajun chicken salad bowl 114
    Greek tuna salad 116
    Potato salad with spinach and chorizo 112
    Pulled pork, rice and kale salad 111
    Refreshing detox salad 104
    Roasted rainbow veggie breakfast
        salad 80
    Roasted rainbow veggie, kale and
        quinoa salad 100
    Simple roasted veggie salad 105
    Tuna, roasted pumpkin and brown rice
        salad 102
    Zesty Greek salad with pulled pork 110
Salted caramel porridge 61
sausages
    Breakfast tray bake 62
    Potato salad with spinach and
        chorizo 112
    Sausage and vegetable pasta bake 136
Sausage and vegetable pasta bake 136
seafood
    Flash-fried squid with rocket and
        pineapple 152
    Mango, coconut and chilli prawns 153
shopping in bulk 8, 10, 18, 21, 30
Silky skin smoothie 95
Simple roasted veggie salad 105

slices
    Choc–marshmallow slice 220
    Corn and ham breakfast slice 77
    Fruity breakfast slice 61
    Lemon and coconut slice 228
    Peppermint–choc slice 232
sloppy joes, Pulled pork and spinach 163
Slow-cooked beef nachos 200
Slow-cooked fish curry with pappadums 161
Slow-cooked lemon pudding 241
Slow-cooked vegetable and tortellini
    soup 126
smoothies 26
    Bright eyes smoothie 86
    Chocolate–raspberry smoothie 87
    Coco–banana bliss smoothie 95
    Coconut rough smoothie 90
    Energising smoothie 96
    Fruit fusion smoothie 90
    Immunity-boosting smoothie 91
    Mango–passionfruit smoothie 97
    Minty coconut smoothie 87
    Peaches and cream smoothie 97
    Peanut butter and jelly smoothie 91
    Raspberry–oat smoothie 94
    Recovery smoothie 94
    Silky skin smoothie 95
    Tropical green smoothie 86
soups
    Beef, lentil and veggie soup 130
    Coconutty pumpkin soup 128
    Slow-cooked vegetable and tortellini
        soup 126
Spicy chicken and corn soup 129
Spiced chicken and roasted rainbow
    veggie tacos 191
Spiced chickpea bowl 108
Spicy broccoli and cheese pikelets 208
Spicy chicken and corn soup 129
spinach
    Baked sweet potatoes with spinach
        and feta 176
    Breakfast tray bake 62
    Buddha bowl 107
    Cajun chicken salad bowl 114
    Cheesy chicken meatballs in tomato
        and spinach sauce 156
    Corn and ham breakfast slice 77
    Ham, spinach and feta pizzas 189
    Open burger with the lot 164
    Potato salad with spinach and
        chorizo 112
    Pulled pork and spinach sloppy
        joes 163
    Roasted rainbow veggie breakfast
        salad 80
    Silky skin smoothie 95
    Slow-cooked vegetable and tortellini
        soup 126
    Tropical green smoothie 86
    Zesty Greek salad with pulled pork 110
    Zucchini and ricotta bake 64
squid: Flash-fried squid with rocket and
    pineapple 152
strawberries
    Fruit fusion smoothie 90
    Peanut butter and jelly smoothie 91

Super-quick ham, cheese and tomato
    quiche 122
Sweet chilli tuna rice paper rolls 123
sweet potatoes 21
    Bacon and egg with veggie hash 67
    Baked sweet potatoes with spinach
        and feta 176
    Breakfast tray bake 62
    Cajun chicken salad bowl 114
    Lentil shepherd's pie 174
    Roasted rainbow veggie breakfast
        salad 80
    Roasted rainbow veggie, kale and
        quinoa salad 100
    Roasted rainbow veggies 37
    Spiced chicken and roasted rainbow
        veggie tacos 191
    Spiced chickpea bowl 108
    Sweet potato and chickpea curry 160
    Sweet potato fries with garlicky dip 207
Sweet potato and chickpea curry 160
Sweet potato fries with garlicky dip 207

T

tacos, Fish, with coleslaw 179
tacos, Spiced chicken and roasted rainbow
    veggie 191
tart, Pumpkin and feta 188
Thai chicken meatloaf 184
The Healthy Mummy 7, 8, 34–35
tofu: Creamy passionfruit and mango ice
    blocks 235
tomatoes
    Baked cheese and tomato risotto 140
    Cheesy chicken meatballs in tomato
        and spinach sauce 156
    Chicken and corn fritters 154
    Chicken burrito bowls 167
    Gourmet scrambled eggs 66
    Greek tuna salad 116
    Ham, spinach and feta pizzas 189
    Hawaiian melts 78
    Hidden veg bolognese 40
    Hidden veg bolognese pie 196
    Hidden veg bolognese potatoes 197
    Lentil shepherd's pie 174
    Mediterranean chicken and vegetable
        pasta 138
    Mexican breakfast wrap 74
    Mushroom and sun-dried tomato mini
        frittatas 73
    Open burger with the lot 164
    Pulled pork and spinach sloppy
        joes 163
    Ratatouille lasagne 135
    Super-quick ham, cheese and tomato
        quiche 122
    Sweet potato and chickpea curry 160
    Tuna and pumpkin mac and cheese 141
    Tuna, roasted pumpkin and brown rice
        salad 102
    Turkey and salad sub 123
    Turkey meatballs and spaghetti 143
    Veggie-loaded fritters 69
    Zesty Greek salad with pulled pork 110
    Zoodles with hidden veg bolognese 144

Tropical green smoothie 86
tuna
    Greek tuna salad 116
    Sweet chilli tuna rice paper rolls 123
    Tuna and pumpkin mac and cheese 141
    Tuna, roasted pumpkin and brown rice
        salad 102
Tuna and pumpkin mac and cheese 141
Tuna, roasted pumpkin and brown rice
    salad 102
Turkey and salad sub 123
Turkey meatballs and spaghetti 143
Turmeric egg and bacon wrap 79

V

Veggie-loaded fritters 69

W

watermelon: Fruit fusion smoothie 90
weight loss 8, 9, 10
wrap, Chicken caesar 119
wrap, Mexican breakfast 74

Z

Zesty Greek salad with pulled pork 110
Zoodles with hidden veg bolognese 144
zucchini
    Bacon and zucchini muffins 72
    Hoisin pork with greens and rice 193
    Lamb and lentil curry 41
    Lamb and lentil curry pasties 199
    Lamb and lentil curry with coriander
        rice 171
    Lamb and lentil curry-stuffed
        zucchini 194
    Mediterranean chicken and vegetable
        pasta 138
    Mini cheese, ham and quinoa
        muffins 212
    Ratatouille lasagne 135
    Roasted rainbow veggie breakfast
        salad 80
    Roasted rainbow veggie, kale and
        quinoa salad 100
    Roasted rainbow veggies 37
    Sausage and vegetable pasta bake 136
    Simple roasted veggie salad 105
    Slow-cooked vegetable and tortellini
        soup 126
    Spiced chicken and roasted rainbow
        veggie tacos 191
    Veggie-loaded fritters 69
    Zoodles with hidden veg
        bolognese 144
    Zucchini and ricotta bake 64
Zucchini and ricotta bake 64

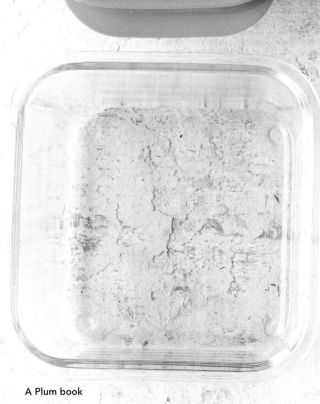

A Plum book

First published in 2019 by
Pan Macmillan Australia Pty Limited
Level 25, 1 Market Street,
Sydney, NSW 2000, Australia

Level 3, 112 Wellington Parade,
East Melbourne, VIC 3002, Australia

Design by Kirby Armstrong
Edited by Rachel Carter
Index by Helena Holmgren
Food photography by Chris Middleton
Additional photography by Steve Brown
Prop and food styling by Lee Blaylock and Vanessa Austin
Food preparation by Caroline Griffiths, Rachael Lane and Sarah Mayoh
Typeset by Megan Ellis
Colour reproduction by Splitting Image Colour Studio
Printed and bound in China by 1010 Printing International Limited

A CIP catalogue record for this book is available from the National Library of Australia.